THE HEALTHY
KNEES BOOK

by Astrid Pujari, M.D., & Nancy Schatz Alton

THE HEALTHY KNEES BOOK

A GUIDE TO WHOLE HEALING FOR OUTDOOR ENTHUSIASTS AND OTHER ACTIVE PEOPLE

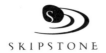

SKIPSTONE

© 2010 by Astrid Pujari, MD, and Nancy Schatz Alton

Published by Skipstone, an imprint of The Mountaineers Books
Printed in the United States of America
First printing 2010
13 12 11 10   5 4 3 2 1

Copy Editor: Joan Gregory
Design: Heidi Smets
Illustrations: Kate Quinby
Cover photograph: © Erik Isakson/Tetra Images/Getty Images

ISBN (paperback) 978-1-59485-013-4
ISBN (ebook) 978-1-59485-404-0

Library of Congress Cataloging-in-Publication Data
Pujari, Astrid, 1971-
  The healthy knees book : a guide to whole healing for outdoor enthusiasts & other active people / by Astrid Pujari, and Nancy Schatz Alton.
      p. cm.
  Includes bibliographical references and index.
  ISBN 978-1-59485-013-4
 1. Knee—Wounds and injuries—Alternative treatment. 2. Knee—Diseases—Alternative treatment. I. Alton, Nancy Schatz, 1970- II. Title.
  RD561.P85 2010
  617.5'82044—dc22

                    2009039543

Skipstone books may be purchased for corporate, educational, or other promotional sales. For special discounts and information, contact our Sales Department at 800-553-4453 or mbooks@mountaineersbooks.org.

Skipstone
1001 SW Klickitat Way, Suite 201
Seattle, Washington 98134
206.223.6303
www.skipstonepress.org
www.mountaineersbooks.org

LIVE LIFE. MAKE RIPPLES.

CONTENTS

(handwritten in margin: 14.36)

(handwritten in margin: June 9/10)

PREFACE

Not long ago, I was about to give a lecture about integrative medicine to a room full of doctors. Before the talk, a man walked up to me. "What's the point of all that holistic, alternative medicine stuff?" he asked. "Don't you have enough to do with just the conventional medicine? How can you possibly have the time to talk with patients about more?"

It's true that most doctors are swamped for time. When I was working in primary care, I had fifteen minutes allotted for each patient. Half of that time was already accounted for—checking previous medical and lab reports, dictating notes, and so forth. By the time I walked into the examination room, I had at most eight minutes to listen to the patient's story, examine her, and determine a solution. That's not much time for a doctor-patient interaction, as I'm sure you know. Is there really time for discussion that goes beyond conventional medicine?

I believe the answer is yes, because I strongly believe that no single paradigm has all the answers. Healing belongs in a much bigger universe than just the Western medicine worldview. How can we expect any one truth—no matter how helpful—to answer all of our questions when it comes to the infinite complexity of human health?

All of this reminds me of the story of the three men trying to describe an elephant. The man at the front said, "An elephant is an animal with a long nose and tusks." The man at the side said, "Elephants are animals with gray skin," while the man at the back said, "The elephant is an animal with wiry hair and a thin tail." Every one of these men was correct—and their perspectives limited all of them. It is only in combining their viewpoints that one begins to see what an elephant really looks like.

The same point applies to human health—which is exactly why it is so important to *integrate* various philosophies of healing and why I now work as an integrative medicine physician. Time and time again, as a primary care doctor, I met people whose problems could not be resolved through conventional Western medicine. It's no wonder that I started looking outside the box. I really wanted to help people, but in order to do that, I had to expand my toolkit.

Which is the point of this book.

Knee pain, as you may know, is a very common reason for people to see their primary care doctors. And rightly so—it makes sense that people would be pretty motivated to have healthy knees, since without them, it is impossible to walk, bend, or play most sports. The only problem is that we doctors usually end up giving our patients pills to take and physical therapy to do, but that doesn't always fix the problem, or it may not be enough. Or perhaps, you don't want to take prescription medication, but you do want to get completely, and permanently, better. So what can you do?

This book seeks to address those questions. In it are some simple, effective techniques to help you expand *your* toolkit in a practical way. We give you a whole host of ideas—from nutrition to acupuncture to yoga to physical therapy to mind–body techniques to stretching exercises—about how to take charge of your knees and your health in a way that addresses the whole person, not just part of you. We also tell you when you should talk to your doctor and what to say when you get there. In fact, your new toolkit may even help your doctor to expand his.

This is, of course, one of my hopes. I believe that the best kinds of healing work on our insides and our outsides at the same time, because as human beings, we don't live in an isolated vacuum but in an interconnected web of life. Every time we take a step to integrate different paradigms of healing for our own good, we help everyone around us to do the same. That is how harmony continues to grow itself—and nothing could be more healing for us, or for our world, than that.

Astrid Pujari, MD, MNIMH
April 2010

ACKNOWLEDGMENTS

In the name of research, I had the good fortune to interview a range of health care specialists. Our conversations were always chock full of compelling information. Just ask my friends and family: I was always talking about the latest interview. These generous practitioners shared both their knowledge and time. Their years of experience have informed the writing of this book, and I am grateful for their willingness to chat with me.

One of my sources was an integral part of the research and writing of this book. I lost count of the number of times I interviewed Wolfgang Brolley, RPT, LMP, owner of Stretch Physical Therapy in Seattle. This physical therapist and massage therapist has a gift for explaining how the body works. His willingness to read rough drafts of chapters also made this book a better read.

Numerous physicians explained the intricacies of the knee, detailing the injuries and conditions that can occur in and around this joint. We discussed knee anatomy; how they diagnose and treat knee pain; and how patients can alleviate their pain. Dr. Rosemary Agostini is a sports medicine specialist and a family practice physician at Group Health Cooperative in Seattle. Dr. M. Pilar Almy, a Seattle-area podiatrist, shared her knowledge of the foot's role in knee problems. Dr. David Belfie is an orthopedic surgeon who practices in Seattle. Dr. Timothy E. Hewett is a professor and director at Cincinnati Children's Hospital Sports Medicine Biodynamics Center. Orthopedic surgeon Lawrence Holland, MD, practices in Seattle. Dr. Chris Wahl is an orthopedic surgeon at the University of Washington in Seattle.

I talked with numerous physical therapists, and their expertise informs several chapters, including "Knee Anatomy 101," "Common Knee Problems," "Your Knees and the Sports You Play," "Stretch Your Body," "Finding a Movement Professional", "Bodyworks", and "Western Medical Interventions." I need to thank Wolfgang Brolley here as well. Ken Cole, PT, COMT, FAAOMPT, CFI, is the managing partner of Olympic Physical Therapy in Renton, Washington. He has designed a specialized motor-control sports medicine program for ground, water, and air athletes for injury prevention and rapid return to activity based on the biomechanical model of the McConnell and North American Institute of Manual Therapy. Annie O'Connor, PT, OCS, Cert. MDT, is the corporate director of Musculoskeletal Practice at the Rehabilitation Institute of Chicago (RIC) and she runs the internal residency-training program for physical therapists at RIC. Mark Looper, PT, MS, COMT, FAAOMPT, is the managing partner of Olympic Physical Therapy of Kirkland, Washington, and principal partner of Seattle-based Olympic Physical Therapy. He has developed a spine stabilization program for both the sporting and nonathletic community. Physical therapist Ellen Roth practices in Seattle. Physical therapist Jane Vess works in the rehabilitation department of St. Agnes Hospital in Baltimore, Maryland.

Several movement professionals, from occupational therapists to exercise specialists, lent their knowledge to Chapter Four: "Stretch Your Body."

Some of them shared exercises, while others talked about how to move your body throughout the day, from setting up a workstation to performing everyday tasks. ACSM-certified personal trainer Sebastian Alery is also a master swim coach and massage therapist. Wolfgang Brolley's knowledge informs this chapter. Barb Mierzwa, OTR/L, is an occupational therapist at Rehabilitation Institute of Washington. Ellen Roth is a Seattle-area physical therapist. Occupational therapist Carolyn Salazar, MS, works at Valley Medical Center Occupational Health Services in Renton, Washington.

Researchers Karen Sherman, PhD, and Daniel Cherkin, PhD, conduct their studies at Group Health Research Institute. We talked about their research on yoga, acupuncture, physical therapy, exercise, chiropractic care, and massage therapy, as well as the mind–body connection and the role of belief in healing.

Several movement professional lent their knowledge to this book, including the chapters "Your Knees and the Sports You Play," "Stretch Your Body," "Finding a Movement Professional," and "Bodyworks." Stott Pilates instructor-trainer Shane Belau is cofounder of Bodycenter Studios, a Pilates studio in Seattle. Valerie Crosby is a certified yoga teacher in Albuquerque, New Mexico. Jennifer Keeler is a certified yoga teacher who runs Yoga Momma at the Phinney Yoga House in Seattle, Washington. Cathy Prescott is a senior teacher and mentor for Integrative Yoga Therapy who lives in Niskayanu, New York. Stott Pilates instructor-trainer Kristi Quinn is a cofounder of Bodycenter Studios, a Pilates studio in Seattle. Marjorie Thompson is the lead instructor and program director of Seattle's Pacific Northwest Ballet's Pilates program, PNBConditioning. Seattle-based Laura Yon-Brooks, MA, LMP, RYT, is a sports medicine professional and yoga teacher who has worked with professional athletes.

Although much of the information in the chapter "Practices for the Mind" comes from coauthor Astrid Pujari, I also spoke with Dr. Herbert Benson of the Benson-Henry Institute for Mind Body Medicine at Massachusetts General Hospital. Dr. Benson was one of the first doctors to connect meditation and Western medicine in the United States.

The "Bodyworks" chapter includes information from several professionals. Occupational therapist and Bowenworks practitioner Kelly Clancy runs BalanceOT, Inc., and the Seattle Center for Structural Medicine, which are both in Seattle. Acupuncturist and hypnotist Randy Clere is also a martial arts master, a shiatsu massage therapist and an NLP practitioner in Seattle. Stephanie Colony is a former Hellerworks practitioner in Seattle. Naturopathic physician and acupuncturist Dr. Kevin Connor works at Seattle Healing Arts. Dr. Lew Estabrook is a Seattle-area chiropractor. Dr. Katie Larkin is a pediatric acupuncturist, an anesthesiologist, and a pain management doctor at Stanford University in California. Feldenkrais practitioner Marsha Novak, GCFP, PT, runs Moving Well Physical Therapy & Movement Education in Seattle. Rolfer Michael Reams practices in Seattle.

Along with the doctors and physical therapists I interviewed for the "Western Medical Interventions" chapter, I talked with psychotherapist Peggy Huddleston. Although surgery is a major medical intervention, there is not much information out there for people hoping to mentally prepare for and recover from operations. Her book *Prepare for Surgery, Heal Faster: A Guide of Mind–Body Techniques* fills this role.

This book wouldn't be in your hands right now without the help of people who haven't studied the amazing knee, as well. My personal support staff kept me going as I wound my way through the intricacies of both the knee and numerous avenues of healing. My husband Chris cheered me on, cooked countless meals, and kept the home and family running smoothly. My daughters Caroline and Elizabeth Annie made me forget about my computer (sometimes by telling me to "turn that off now"), which was a welcome reprieve. My love of the written word started long ago, thanks to my immediate family; thanks to my entire extended family (Altons and Schatzs) for continuing to foster that addiction and support me in my endeavors. My friends lent their ears and gave me much needed assistance all year long: Mary, Linda, Jen, Beth, Julie, Marie, Kirsten, Dave, my "editor friends," and the entire St. John crew.

Thanks to my editors: Joan Gregory, editor extraordinaire, helped clarify my words and work. Mary Metz saw the book through its final stages. The idea for this holistic health guide series comes from Kate Rogers at The Mountaineers Books and Skipstone. Thank you for giving me this opportunity and walking me through the writing of my first books.

Lastly, thanks to my coauthor Dr. Astrid Pujari. I am grateful for your clear and joyful presence, as well as your impressive knowledge about the human body and holistic health care.

—Nancy Schatz Alton

I, too, wish to extend my sincere thanks and appreciation to all those who shared their time, knowledge, and expertise to make this book possible. A special thanks to my coauthor, Nancy Schatz Alton, who has an amazing gift for distilling complicated information into an easy, fun-to-read presentation. And thanks to you, the reader, for being willing to explore the horizons of this new medicine, which combines the best of every tradition.

—Astrid Pujari, MD

INTRODUCTION

MOVING YOUR BODY IS SIMPLE as long as its major joints are in excellent condition. Your knees, which house your body's largest joints, help you sit, skip, run, leap, and pivot with absolute ease. Essential to efficient locomotion, they make everyday actions possible. Without a thought, you can squat in your garden to pull weeds or kneel on the floor to pick up your child. You can ride your bike in the morning, take a weekend climb with your friends, or go backcountry skiing in the winter.

Your knees make spectacular tasks doable, too. They need to be in good working order to complete a marathon, climb Mount Denali, or finish the Seattle-to-Portland bike ride. Of course, lots of us just want a simple Saturday hike with our family, a weekly soccer game, or a part in the annual 3-on-3 March Madness basketball competition.

It pays to keep our knees happy. These shock-absorbing joints take a lot of abuse in the course of a lifetime. Every year, knee injuries send roughly 9.5 million people in the United States to an orthopedic specialist's office.

Although the knee is quite durable, it is one of our body's most complex structures. Linking the two longest bones of the body—the thigh and shin—each knee joint is formed by bones, ligaments, tendons, muscles, fluid-filled sacs, and cartilage. This hinge joint also rotates, and although this extra mobility helps us move, it also makes knee injuries more prevalent.

Outside the examining room, there are measures you can take to keep your knees strong and to prevent injuries. When trauma occurs, you can alleviate the hurt through self-care. Although there are surgical repairs for several knee injuries, rehabilitation after any surgery is vital. Many knee problems have nonsurgical solutions, with numerous alternatives for strengthening and healing your knees. Being a thoughtful consumer of knee pain prevention and remedies is helpful.

Taking anti-inflammatory pain medication is just one option for dealing with occasional knee pain, just as seeing a physical therapist is one of several ways of approaching a chronic knee problem. Even though you rely on your sports medicine doctor regarding your torn ACL, you are ultimately in charge of your own healing. Whether you have daily pain or bouts of pain due to osteoarthritis or the occasional achy knees during steep hiking descents, you don't need to rely on just one system of health care. Medical care today offers a broad range of options: Western medicine, complementary treatments, alternative care, Eastern practices, and more. When you're looking for relief from pain, you can choose from a broad array of healing practices.

Picture the various types of therapies available to you as spokes on a wheel. Imagine yourself standing on the hub of that wheel. You can select any combination of therapies, or spokes, from this big wheel. Massage therapy might be a complementary addition to physical therapy. Acupuncture can provide post-operative pain relief.

In this book, we take a holistic approach to healing. First, we'll look closely at your knees, learning about each part and how it functions. Next, we'll talk about the knees' most common injuries and chronic pain problems. The following chapters explore various avenues to healing. Instead of considering only one fix, we'll discuss numerous remedies. One or more of these therapies might help you find relief from your knee pain. We've compiled information from medical specialists, physical therapists, yoga and fitness instructors, bodyworks practitioners, nutritionists, and herbalists. Since our lives move at warp speed these days, *The Healthy Knee Book: A Guide to Whole Healing for Outdoor Enthusiasts & Other Active People* offers simple solutions for the time-crunched reader.

The information in this book is based on the research and experience of the authors. It is not intended to be a substitute for consulting with your physician or healthcare provider. Any attempt to diagnose and treat an illness should be done under the direction of a health care professional. The publisher and authors are not responsible for any adverse effects or consequences resulting from the use of any of the suggestions, preparations, or procedures discussed in this book.

1   KNEE ANATOMY 101

WE'VE ALL HEARD THAT KNOWLEDGE IS POWER. When it comes to your aching knees, this saying takes on special meaning. Understanding knee anatomy helps you navigate your road to healing. Think about your biking trip through rural France. Although it wasn't absolutely necessary to have a working knowledge of the French language, it sure made the journey easier.

Medical terminology can sound like a foreign language. Regardless, talking to your care provider is easier if you can picture how your knee works. Perusing the miles of online material on knee problems becomes a simpler task. And if words such as *adductors* and *gastrocnemius* roll off your tongue during conversations, people at social gatherings may even mistake you for a doctor.

All kidding aside, learning the technical jargon about the knee will help you create a plan for treating your knee ailment.

BONES 1, 2, 3, AND 4

Just four bones comprise the knee. The top bone is the *femur*, or *thigh-bone*, which is the longest bone in your body. The main weight-bearing bone below the femur is the *tibia*, or *shinbone*, which happens to be the second-longest bone in your body. Toward the outside of the leg—or to the lateral side, as doctors like to say—the *fibula* bone resides next to the tibia. Between the tibia and fibula is an *interosseous membrane*. As weight bears down on the tibia, the fibers of this membrane transfer forces to the fibula, which then takes on a small percentage of the load.

The oval-shaped *patella* is the bone we all think of as the *kneecap*. It is quite small, yet thick. In fact, the patella has the thickest cartilage of your entire body; this protects it from the forces traveling through your knee as you move. The patella itself resides within a space called the *trochlear groove*—a space between the two rounded ends, or *condyles*—of the femur bone. To get an even more distinct picture of kneecap anatomy, let's talk about tendons and ligaments.

TENDONS AND LIGAMENTS

Tendons and ligaments are essentially connective tissues. As a rule, *tendons* connect muscles to bones and *ligaments* connect bone to bone. Both tendons and ligaments consist of strands of elastic proteins. When you come to a quick stop while skiing, your ligaments prevent your bones from moving too far. Tendons are more elastic, helping your muscles move. Don't be fooled by this flexibility: tendons are actually stronger than steel.

The patella, or kneecap, lives within a tendon. Called the *patellar tendon*, this tendon attaches the quadriceps muscles on the front of your thigh and envelops your patella. As the patellar tendon reaches your shinbone, it inserts into the *tibial tuberosity*. If you bend your knee, you might glimpse your tibial tuberosity: use your fingertips to feel for a slight, bony bulge just below your kneecap. In anatomical jargon, the patellar tendon-kneecap combination is a *sesamoid bone*. This term simply means a bone resides inside a tendon, helping you move with as little friction as possible. Your kneecap-patellar tendon is the largest of the sesamoid bones in your body. The knobby bone you feel on the outer side of your wrist near your pinky and on your palm, called the *pisiform*, is also a sesamoid bone.

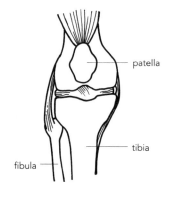

1.1. Basic Knee Anatomy

Keeping Motion in Check

As you jump and land while going for that slam-dunk, your four knee ligaments keep each knee's motion in check. First up are two collateral ligaments that sit outside your knee joint. The *lateral collateral ligament*, or *LCL*, is on the outer side of the leg, connecting the femur to the fibula. The *medial collateral ligament*, or *MCL*, is on the inside part of the leg, connecting the femur to the tibia. Both the LCL and MCL stop your leg from bending sideways. To see this in action, hold up your hand. With a finger from your opposite hand, try to push any finger to

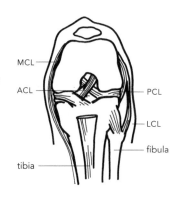

1.2. Knee Ligaments (front of left knee)

one side and then the other side. Notice the limits on your finger's range of motion. Ligaments on the sides of your fingers that are similar in nature to your LCL and MCL ligaments prevent your fingers from bending too far side to side. If you stand up and try to bend your leg outward or inward, the LCL and MCL stop your bones from bending too far.

The last ligament pair includes the famed *anterior cruciate ligament,* or *ACL,* and the nearly forgotten *posterior cruciate ligament,* or *PCL.* If you stand and cross your right leg in front of your left leg, your right leg is an example of the ACL. It goes from the back bottom of the femur (thighbone), comes forward and across the knee joint, and attaches to the front top of the tibia (shinbone). The PCL crosses the ACL, coming from the front bottom of the femur, going back and across the knee joint, and attaching to the back top of the tibia. Both the ACL and PCL act like brakes on the lower leg. The ACL stops the tibia from sliding too far forward, while the PCL keeps the tibia from sliding too far back, both in relation to the femur. Both ligaments help stabilize the knee, while also giving it some rotational ability.

CARTILAGE

Cartilage covers the ends of most bones in our bodies, including our knee bones. Called *articular cartilage,* it looks like the white, shiny cartilage at the ends of chicken bones. You can put your fingernail in it because it is soft. Orthopedic surgeons compare it to a Teflon coating in a nonstick pan; this tough, resistant connective tissue absorbs shock and prevents bone damage. Articular cartilage resists the sheer force of two bone surfaces gliding over each other.

A second kind of cartilage in the knee also helps to absorb shock, ease movement, and disperse weight. Called the *meniscal cartilage,* it has a spongy, rubber band-like texture. Your knee joint has two meniscal cartilages: the *medial meniscus* near the inside of your knee, and the *lateral meniscus* near the outside of your knee. The meniscal cartilage makes the joint congruent, mating a curved surface with a flat surface. The femur bone ends in two rounded condyles, or prominences. However, the top of the tibia bone—referred to as the *tibial plateau*—is relatively flat. The end surfaces of the tibia and femur sit within this meniscal cartilage, which makes for almost frictionless, smooth actions. If you were to look down at the interior of the knee joint, you would note that each meniscus is high on the outside, tapering down on each end, with each meniscus making a nice C-shaped curve.

MUSCLES

Your muscles help move your knees. They initiate movement and are yet another body part that keeps your knee from moving too far. Think of your muscles as levers and pulleys, working underneath your skin to make everyday actions possible. Working mostly in pairs, muscles move in two ways: lengthening (*eccentric motion*) and shortening (*concentric motion*). Consider the biceps muscles on your arm. If you are doing a biceps curl, the biceps muscles are shortening, or contracting, as they work; this is concentric motion. Next, you grab a heavy weight and slowly lower that weight. Your biceps muscles are still working or else you would drop that heavy weight on your foot. Now the muscles are lengthening, or eccentrically contracting. Your leg muscles move in a similar fashion as you bend and straighten your lower leg.

The muscles that help move and stabilize your knee are numerous. It's useful to know about a handful of these muscles and their roles in knee health. Some of the muscles are two-jointed muscles, meaning they cross two joints: the hip and the knee. Some of the muscles start all the way up in the lower back. This means that both the lower back and the hip and some of their associated muscles can affect your knees and lead to injury.

Muscles Bend and Straighten the Leg

Let's start with the thigh muscles. Put a hand on the front of each thigh: your quadriceps muscles are located here. They are called the *quadriceps muscles* because there are four of them: the *vastus lateralis,* the *vastus intermedius,* the *vastus medialis,* and the *rectus femoris.* These extensors of the knee take your bent knee and straighten it. All of the vastus muscles are one-joint muscles, while the rectus femoris crosses both the hip and the knee. All of the four quadriceps muscles attach on the femur bone, coalesce together, and feed into the patellar tendon.

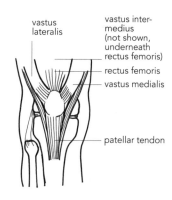

1.3. Quadriceps Muscles
(front of right knee)

Now place your hands on the backs of your thighs. Your *hamstring muscles* are here. These muscles take your straight leg and bend it. Coming down from the hip to the knee, these three muscles are the *biceps femoris,* the *semimembranosus,* and the *semitendinosus.* The hamstring muscles don't come together the way the quadriceps muscles do. Instead, each muscle attaches separately to the knee joint. The semitendinosus joins the *sartorius* and *gracilis,* and then attaches to the tibia on the inside part of the knee in a bundle of tendons called the *pes anserinus.* As a group, these three muscles help the knee both flex and rotate inwards. Pes anserinus

KEEP YOUR FEET HAPPY

Your foot is the first part of your body to hit the ground, the very beginning of the kinetic chain, translating up the entire leg all the way to your backbone. During pronation, your heel touches the pavement as your foot flexes in and downward to adapt to the floor and absorb shock. Later, during supination, your foot rolls outwards and stiffens, giving you a rigid, level support to push your foot and body forward.

Pronation and supination are part of your gait, or the way you walk. If you over-pronate, meaning there is too much of an internal or downward movement, this rotates your shinbone inward, which can negatively affect your knee.

If you over-supinate, your gait is much more jarring, which can lead to arthritis. Someone with flat feet—meaning there are no upward arches on the bottom of her feet—expends more energy moving because her feet lack that rigid support that naturally pushes her forward.

If you are suffering from a knee problem, the root of your injury could be your gait. Since any of these foot issues can lead to knee problems, it makes sense to have a professional look at your gait. Your doctor can watch you walk, but he may send you to a podiatrist for further analysis. Orthotics—inserts for your shoes—are often the solution for gait issues. Sometimes orthotics will need to be custom-made. Often, though, your regular doctor or a podiatrist will suggest over-the-counter orthotics. Dr. Pilar Almy, a Seattle-area podiatrist, recommends visiting shoe specialty shops to buy orthotics, as opposed to purchasing them at your local pharmacy. At an athletics shop, an outdoor store, or a running gear shop, a clerk versed in your sport and footwear will have you try on several styles of shoes, watching your gait as you jump, hike, or run. Often stores will have treadmills, so they can watch your gait while you run or walk. Besides guiding you to specific footwear, a clerk can point out suitable orthotics for your gait issues. Dr. Almy recommends the following brands to her patients:

- Superfeet
- Sole
- Biosoft
- Quick-Stride
- Lyncos

Even if you don't have any pronation or supination issues during your everyday life, participating in athletics may exaggerate a minor gait defect. This is why being professionally fitted for your athletic shoes is a good idea.

means "goosefoot" because as these muscles join together they look like the three toes of a goose's foot.

Move your hands to the insides of your thighs to feel your *adductor muscles*. Three of these muscles attach to the femur bone, so they don't directly affect the knee joint.

Only one calf muscle directly affects your knee, the *gastrocnemius*. This main calf muscle attaches above the knee at the femur bone and extends all the way to your heel. To feel your gastrocnemius, run your hand behind your knee and down the back of your lower leg. Although this muscle primarily flexes the foot, it also flexes the knee joint. When you stand, jump, walk, or run, you can thank your gastrocnemius.

The *popliteus* and *plantaris* muscles are small muscles located behind your knee. Both of these muscles help flex the knee, and the popliteus assists with unlocking the knee and turning the leg.

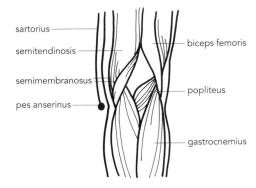

1.4. Hamstring Muscles (back of right knee)

Picture Saran Wrap

Next, place your hands on the sides of your thighs. Your *iliotibial bands* are here. Nicknamed the *IT band*, this swath of muscle extends all the way from your hip to your shinbone. Picture the IT band as a large sheet of Saran Wrap. This swath of connective tissue starts on the outer curve of your pelvic bone, moves down the hip and outer leg, goes past the knee, and then inserts into the tibia at a spot called *Gerdy's tubercle* (close to the tibial tuberosity, where the patellar tendon or ligament inserts). When muscles bend your knee, the IT band slides back, becoming a knee flexor. When the thigh muscles extend your knee, this muscle sheet goes forward, becoming a knee extender.

Bursa

Bursae are fluid-filled sacs that cushion joints. They help lessen friction and wear-and-tear between body parts, including bones, muscles, and tendons. Two bursae that may cause knee pain are the *prepatellar bursa* and the *pes anserine bursa.* Your prepatellar bursa is located on top of the kneecap. The pes anserine bursa is situated roughly two to five centimeters down from the knee joint on the inside of the shinbone and underneath the pes anserinus tendon.

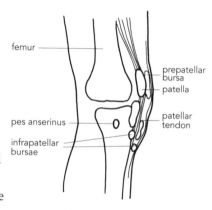

1.5. Bursa (inside of left knee)

YOUR PIVOTING HINGE JOINTS

The knee is a hinge joint: picture a door opening and closing. The knee extends or straightens and flexes or bends. Although most hinge joints move in just one plane, the knee can also rotate. Although knees are quite durable, this extra mobility means the knee is less stable than a simple hinge joint. The knee's motion is also dependent on soft connective tissues, including ligaments, tendons, and cartilage.

Your knee joint also has a *synovial capsule,* which is similar to a water balloon located above and under the kneecap and surrounding the joint.

This tough joint capsule provides protection for the *synovial lining,* which produces and secretes fluid that lubricates and feeds the knee joint. This fat- and protein-rich fluid is continually absorbed into your knee's cartilage. Think about adding grease to your bicycle chain: the grease helps the links move easily along the gears and lessens the wear and tear on the chain. The synovial capsule and its fluid help the knee parts glide smoothly over each other in an almost friction-free manner.

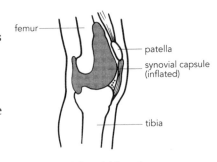

femur
patella
synovial capsule (inflated)
tibia

1.6. Synovial Capsule

THE KNEE BONE CONNECTS TO THE...

Like all of the body's individual parts, the knee doesn't exist in a vacuum. The knee links to the shinbone, the ankle, and the foot, as well as to the hip, the buttocks, and the back, all the way up to the brain. When we think about knee injuries, it's important to look at the rest of the body. Part of this relates to how our body's alignment affects the knee, and part of this relates to how the brain connects to our whole body. In the bigger picture, this mind–body connection links up to the rest of our lives, including how we react to pain, our past and current life experiences, and our belief systems. Two people can have similar knee conditions that show up on an MRI, but only one of them may experience pain.

We'll talk about these connections throughout this book, and it's good to keep them in mind as we discuss common problems that affect our knees. While treating the knee is dependent on a specific diagnosis at times, knee pain is also about management. Because each person is unique, solutions to a knee condition can take countless forms.

2 COMMON KNEE PROBLEMS

IF WE FALL ON THE COURT—be it volleyball, basketball, or any number of fast-paced game arenas—we know to check our knees for signs of injury. Our knees scream loudly when seriously injured, popping and making the hurt known loud and clear. When in agony from a damaged knee, we don't hesitate to visit the local emergency room or our primary care doctor.

Less-persistent knee conditions don't get as much attention. We tend to ignore the occasional twinge, or the fact that our knee has started hurting during longer runs. We pay no attention to the clicking or grinding sounds our knees make as we climb the stairs.

Perhaps, however, your knees have caught your attention lately. You aren't running as much. You sat on the bench for half of last night's basketball game instead of playing. Your climbing club scheduled an ascent this weekend, but you bowed out. Why? Because your knee hurts.

You want to know why your knee hurts. More importantly, you want to play your favorite sports, participate in your favorite activities, and go about your daily routines without worrying about your knees.

Read on to learn about the most common knee problems. When we you know why your knee hurts, you can address the cause of the pain. If an athletic trauma sends you immediately to the ER, understanding your injury will help you take charge of your recovery.

RED FLAG SYMPTOMS

When knee pain flares up, be aware of possible "red flag symptoms." These are warning signs that alert your doctor to serious problems associated with knee pain. In fact, your doctor's first responsibility is to make sure you have no red flag symptoms, ruling out medical conditions that need immediate treatment. If you are experiencing knee pain along with any of the following symptoms, see your doctor or visit an emergency room as soon as possible.

- You can't walk—that is, you can't bear weight on the knee.
- Your knee locks with movement, or buckles or gives out.
- Your knee is deformed, out of joint, or out of place.
- Your knee pain is severe and/or lasts for more than a few days.
- You experience severe swelling and/or a hot, red knee, and/or you have a fever.
- Your knee pain wakes you up at night.

PATELLOFEMORAL (KNEECAP) PAIN

Symptoms: Pain around the kneecap? Pain above the kneecap where the patellar tendon inserts into the femur or thighbone? These are symptoms of what specialists refer to as *patellofemoral pain.* It may hurt more with certain activities, including athletic pursuits, during squatting activities such as gardening, while hiking downhill, or while walking down stairs. The pain is worse after sitting for long periods. Other symptoms include a popping, clicking, or grinding sound when your knee moves, as well as general pain or tenderness in the knee. (If your knee makes similar sounds, but you have no pain, there is no need to worry.)

Explanation: Patellofemoral pain is really a description of pain and not a diagnosis. *Patellofemoral* describes both the kneecap and where the kneecap tendon inserts into the femur or thighbone. If you are hurting in this locale, your doctor may call this pain one of three things: *patellofemoral pain* or *syndrome, anterior knee pain,* or *chondromalacia patella (CMP).*

CMP, however, is not the same as patellofemoral pain or anterior knee pain. If an orthopedic surgeon looks under the surface of your kneecap during surgery and sees the articular cartilage is softening, this is technically CMP. This condition is often a precursor to osteoarthritis. Over time, many doctors have started labeling knee pain as CMP, even if there is no evidence of softening articular cartilage. Ask your doctor what she means if she says you have CMP. Does she really mean you have patellofemoral syndrome or anterior knee pain, not CMP?

Causes: Generally, patellofemoral and anterior knee pain signify an injury in and around the kneecap-femoral structures. This problem can result simply from the way you move your body. For example, while landing from a layup during basketball, your knee will go into a knock-knee position, meaning the knee goes in, and the lower leg goes back out toward the foot.

Poor anatomical alignment can cause your kneecap to tilt when you move. Sometimes an anatomical imbalance will cause the patella to track to the outside of the groove it normally resides in. One common cause occurs when the *vastus medialis*, which pulls the kneecap medially, is weaker than the muscles pulling the kneecap laterally. Physical therapists sometimes recommend strengthening the vastus medialis for patellofemoral pain. Another common cause is weak muscles around your knee, including the quadriceps, the inner thigh muscles, the *gluteus medius* muscles in the buttocks, abdominal core, and pelvic floor muscles. Perhaps poor anatomical alignment causes your kneecap to tilt when you move.

Often this condition is an overuse injury: runners and skiers often suffer from it. Tight hamstrings may also lead to anterior knee pain. Obesity is another risk factor. Young female athletes tend to suffer from this condition, as well. Other factors may include other anatomical issues, biomechanical issues (such as how the foot moves, which affects knee motion), and cyclical hormonal fluctuations that affect soft tissues in the knee.

Some studies show that women are more likely than men to suffer from this type of knee pain. Different theories try to explain the reason behind these statistics; some of these theories are discussed in the "Females and the ACL" box later in this chapter. Other reasons may be the stresses of pregnancy and/or women's tendencies to have knock-knees (meaning the knees turn inward). Women generally have wider pelvises, so the

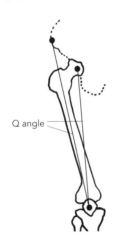

Q angle

2.1. Q Angle

angle of the femur bone goes down and in farther than in men. This may increase the tendency of the patella to pull out of its groove. If your doctor mentions your "Q angle," this is what he is talking about. The Q angle is simply a way to measure how your body aligns between your pelvis, leg, and foot.

Treatment: If you have minor, infrequent patellofemoral pain or CMP, use the "Rest, Ice, Compression, Elevation" method described in the box "R.I.C.E.: Knee Injury Self-Care," on page 37. Until your knee feels better, you may need to avoid the activities that bother it the most, such as hiking, walking down stairs, skiing, running, and sitting for long periods of time.

Upcoming chapters in this book describe various treatments and therapies you apply to your knee. These include the following:

- To ease stiffness and pain and to reduce inflammation, take over-the-counter (OTC) oral non-steroidal anti-inflammatory drugs (NSAIDs), such as aspirin, naproxen, or ibuprofen. You can also use acetaminophen to relieve pain, although it won't reduce inflammation. See Chapter 9 to learn about medications.
- A meditation practice, massage therapy, chiropractic care, and/or acupuncture may help relieve pain as well. See Chapter 6 to learn how meditation can alter your experience of pain; see Chapter 7 for information about bodyworks such as massage or acupuncture.
- A movement practice such as yoga, tai chi, or the Alexander Technique may help strengthen your surrounding muscles, preventing future bouts of pain. Stretching and strengthening the surrounding muscles and your buttocks, core, and pelvic floor muscles will also help. Chapter 5

describes various movement therapies, while Chapter 4 illustrates numerous simple stretches for your knee.

- Changing your diet can ease inflammation from your injury; see Chapter 8 for more information.

If your patellofemoral pain begins limiting your activities too much and the pain seems to be getting worse, visit your primary care provider or a sports medicine physician. Your doctor can confirm your diagnosis. Often she will prescribe a physical therapy rehabilitation program, even if you are suffering from a specific CMP diagnosis. A physical therapist can identify the sources of any knee imbalances, such as alignment issues and weak muscles, and then work on those issues. A physical therapist can help retrain your movement practices, so you are no longer putting undue pressure on your knee.

The physical therapist might have you wear a knee brace that stops and holds the patella in place. Instead of a brace, your physical therapist can teach you how to tape your knee with a method called *McConnell taping*. You'll need to strengthen the quadriceps muscles, especially the VMO, or *vastus medialis oblique* muscle, which is a small part of a quadriceps muscle that inserts into the kneecap. It's also important to work on stretching all the hamstring and quadriceps muscles, making sure these muscles are flexible.

If you have CMP, your doctor may prescribe glucosamine and chondroitin sulfate supplements (see Chapter 8 for information about diets and supplements). CMP may require surgery if small pieces of articular cartilage break loose and become stuck in your knee joint. If your knee locks or you have severe knee pain due to loose articular cartilage—called *loose bodies*—a surgeon can remove these loose bodies during a debridement operation.

R.I.C.E.: KNEE INJURY SELF-CARE

Your knee hurts. It aches after a long day of gardening or it feels out-of-whack after shooting hoops or running hills. The pain doesn't warrant a doctor's visit right now, but how should you care for your knee? Most medical professionals point to the acronym *R.I.C.E.* R.I.C.E. stands for:

- **Rest**: Avoid activities that make your knee hurt. Relative rest usually applies to knee pain. Participate in your daily activities but stop doing anything that causes your knee to cry out in pain. Motion can help promote healing as long as the motion does not cause pain.
- **Ice**: Apply ice. A bag of frozen peas or ice cubes covers the knee better than does an ice pack. On the first day, ice the injury for roughly fifteen minutes every hour or few hours. Keep icing your knee frequently for the next few days.
- **Compression**: Gently compress your knee with a knee brace. Buy a brace at your local pharmacy. Some doctors suggest avoiding Ace bandages, as they are difficult to wrap correctly.
- **Elevation**: Elevate your knee with a pillow so it is at the same level as your heart or above it. Do this as often as possible, while sitting or lying down.

To learn about over-the-counter (OTC) medications that may ease pain, turn to Chapter 9.

MCL & ACL INJURIES

Symptoms: While MCL injuries are the most common ligament problem, sometimes they can go undiagnosed. You may hobble around for a week or two and start to feel better, never visiting a doctor for the problem. Symptoms include pain or inflammation on the inside of your knee. Your knee may hurt if you sleep with your knees one atop another (place a pillow between them to relieve this discomfort). Often you won't know immediately that you injured your MCL. With a more significant injury, the inside of your knee may hurt more, you may have swelling, or your knee may become unstable.

If you tear your ACL, you will usually know immediately. You might hear a pop and feel severe pain or even a snapping sensation. Your knee will probably swell within a few hours of the accident. Symptoms include pain and your leg giving out when you try to put weight on it.

Explanation: Out of the four ligaments that support the knee and connect its bones, the MCL and ACL are much more likely to become strained or torn. The MCL connects the femur, or thighbone, to the tibia, or shinbone, on the inside of each leg. Inside of the knee, the ACL starts at the back bottom of the femur, crosses the knee, and connects to the front top of the tibia. Both of these ligaments keep motion in check. The MCL stops the leg from moving too far side to side while the ACL stops the shinbone from sliding too far forward. Ligament injuries are

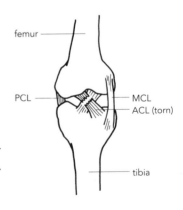

2.2. Tear of ACL (front of right knee)

classified by degrees: 1 is a sprain, 2 is a partial tear, and 3 is a complete tear. Usually an MCL injury is a grade 1 or a low-grade 2. ACL injuries are usually farther along the spectrum, often resulting in a complete tear, although it is possible to strain your ACL.

Causes: An MCL sprain or tear usually requires some contact trauma. When the knee is hit on the outside, the inner top part of the leg can be forced too far in as the foot moves out. Sports such as football, soccer, and skiing are linked to MCL sprains or tears. Still, complete MCL tears are rare. If an MCL tears, often another ligament will tear, usually the ACL.

Although many sports doctors believe the MCL suffers from injury more often, physicians usually diagnose ACL injuries more often. The ACL is usually a noncontact injury, although it is often sports-related. It can happen when the foot remains fixed but the leg keeps moving. Pivoting around a fixed foot or landing from a jump can cause an ACL strain or tear. People hurt their ACL most often during cutting sports, where they change directions quickly, or slow down quickly after moving fast. Examples of cutting sports include football, soccer, basketball, lacrosse, and volleyball. Any sport that requires twisting over a fixed foot can also lead to ACL pain, including skiing.

Treatment: Typical MCL injuries heal within six weeks. As we noted, MCL injuries sometimes go undiagnosed. If you think you have an MCL injury but the pain is minor, use the R.I.C.E. method to take care of yourself (see the box "R.I.C.E.: Knee Injury Self-Care" on page 37). Avoid physical endeavors that cause pain, but go about your normal activities. You should still visit your doctor to confirm the diagnosis.

Upcoming chapters in this book describe various treatments and therapies you can use to address an MCL injury. These include the following:

- Take OTC NSAIDs to relieve pain and reduce inflammation, or take acetaminophen for pain relief. See Chapter 9 to learn about these and other medications.
- Meditation or acupuncture may relieve pain. See Chapter 6 to learn how meditation can alter your experience of pain; see Chapter 7 for information about bodyworks therapies such as acupuncture.
- As you heal, strengthen your surrounding leg muscles through stretches and exercises. A movement therapy such as Pilates or the Feldenkrais Method can also strengthen these muscles. Chapter 4 illustrates numerous stretches for your knee, and Chapter 5 describes various movement therapies.
- Changing your diet can ease inflammation from your injury; see Chapter 8 for more information.

If pain from your MCL injury has you avoiding everyday tasks, or there is swelling, instability, trouble bending the knee, or it doesn't seem to be healing, see your doctor or a sports medicine physician. You may need crutches or a brace to keep the knee immobilized as much as possible. A physical therapy strength-training program may be necessary. Your physical therapist will help you strengthen the MCL's surrounding muscles and increase your knee's range of motion. An MCL injury rarely requires surgery. A partial tear that won't heal with proper treatment may need surgery; a complete tear, especially if more than one ligament is involved, might also call for surgical intervention.

Unlike MCL sprains and tears, ACL tears are most often surgically repaired. See your doctor or a sports medicine physician; he can diagnose your ACL injury level. Although ACL reconstructive surgeries have a more than 80 percent success rate, surgery isn't always necessary. If you only partially tear your ACL, for example, surgery may not be necessary. Of the roughly 200,000 Americans who completely tear their ACL every year, about half of these patients have a surgical reconstruction of their ACL. For more information on the factors that lead a patient to the operating table, turn to Chapter 9. Whether or not you opt for a surgical repair, you will need to take part in physical rehabilitation after an ACL injury.

If you do not have surgery, physical therapy is vital. The hamstring muscles will need to be strong and responsive to help replace lost ACL function. Your physical therapist may have you wear a brace to keep your leg as immobile as possible while you heal. An exercise regimen will work to strengthen all the muscles surrounding the knee joint and help increase your knee's range of motion. Self-care for a minor ACL injury is the same as self-care for an MCL injury (see above). Avoid high-risk activities that could further damage your knee, such as jumping, cutting, pivoting, or suddenly slowing down or stopping.

If you opt for surgery to repair a torn ACL, post-surgical physical therapy is vital. Physical therapy often focuses on learning how to move your body correctly while participating in sporting and leisure activities. After surgery, some patients have trouble using their muscles effectively, so physical therapy will teach the person how to work those muscles again. Electrical stimulation along with an exercise program can help train the muscles. Physical therapy exercises will also help increase the knee's range of motion. It can take up to a year to recover completely from ACL surgery.

Sometimes more than one ligament will become strained or torn. If both the MCL and the ACL are injured, your surgeon will wait until the MCL is healed, and then operate on the ACL. Often, if more than one ligament is injured, the ligaments have a harder time healing; then one or both of the ligaments will need to be surgically repaired.

MENISCAL INJURIES

Symptoms: Meniscal tear symptoms may include joint tenderness, knee pain, swelling, and less-than-smooth knee movement. Do you hear a clicking or feel a catching or a sensation of giving way as your knee moves? Squatting or walking either up or down stairs may hurt. Your knee may lock up, or you might not be able to fully straighten or bend your knee. Significant meniscus tears can lead to loss of frictionless (smooth) knee motion, and eventually lead to osteoarthritis.

Explanation: The meniscus—the cushioning cartilage between your femur and your tibia bones—becomes worn by the stress and sheer of everyday movements and athletics. A torn meniscus simply means there is a disruption or wear of this cartilage.

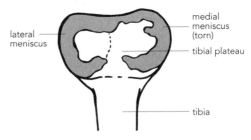

2.3. Medial Meniscal Tear

Causes: Younger people who have meniscal tears and visit the doctor because of the pain usually have a story about how they tore their meniscus. Often the injury occurred during a weight-bearing activity—such as skiing, soccer, basketball, football—with the knee pivoting over a fixed foot. For athletes, it's not uncommon for a meniscal tear to take place alongside injuries to both the MCL and ACL. This is called the "the unhappy triad." Football and soccer players often suffer from this trio of injuries, which often occurs after a player takes a direct hit to the outside of his knee.

If you live long enough, eventually your meniscus will tear. "It functions great for probably the first thirty or forty years, until we are supposed to be eaten by lions," says Dr. Chris Wahl, an orthopedic surgeon at the University of Washington in Seattle. People over the age of forty with meniscus tears usually have no idea how it happened. Often the tear happens over time, due to simple wear and tear. Repetitive squatting motions such as gardening can add to the problem. Often a person with a meniscus tear also has osteoarthritis, which comes from general wear and tear on the knee and can affect both the meniscus and the articular cartilage.

MRI is a very sensitive imaging modality that can discern even mild changes in the quality of meniscus cartilage. "If you carefully reviewed a hundred MRIs of people at age thirty who have no knee symptoms, roughly 25 percent will have some evidence of a meniscus tear," says Dr. Wahl. "And if you take the same number of MRIs of people at age seventy, about 90 percent of them will have MRI evidence of a meniscus tear." Having an MRI that shows a meniscus tear doesn't necessarily mean the tear is the cause of knee pain. Another knee problem may be causing your symptoms.

Treatment: Always book an appointment with your doctor or a sports medicine physician to confirm your diagnosis. Use the R.I.C.E. method to alleviate symptoms (see the box "R.I.C.E.: Knee Injury Self-Care" on page 37).

Upcoming chapters in this book describe various treatments and therapies you can use to address a meniscal injury. These include the following:

▪ Use OTC NSAIDs for swelling and pain relief or acetaminophen to relieve pain. See Chapter 9 to learn about these and other medications.

- Strengthening your surrounding muscles can alleviate the pressure on your meniscus. Stretch your muscles and exercise as often as possible. Try a movement therapy such as yoga, Pilates, the Alexander Technique, or the Feldenkrais Method to strengthen your entire leg and promote proper knee movement. Chapter 4 illustrates numerous exercises and stretches for your knees, and Chapter 5 describes various movement therapies.
- Meditation, hypnotherapy, massage therapy, or acupuncture may alleviate pain. See Chapter 6 to learn how meditation can alter your experience of pain; see Chapter 7 for information about bodyworks therapies such as massage and acupuncture.
- You also can eliminate foods from your diet that promote inflammation; see Chapter 8 for more information.

Your doctor may recommend crutches or fit you with a brace to help keep your knee immobilized, promoting healing and allowing you to participate in more of your favorite activities. Your doctor might also recommend a physical therapist. A physical therapy rehabilitation program will look at the mechanical issues that affect your meniscus. Does the way you move your body cause more meniscal pain? An exercise program will help your knee regain any lost range of motion and strengthen the surrounding muscles.

Younger people without osteoarthritis may need knee arthroscopy to repair their meniscus if symptoms persist. In this procedure, a miniature camera is inserted through a small incision, and the surgeon trims or repairs the tear. Even with an MRI of a torn meniscus, it's important to rule out other sources of knee pain before undergoing an operation. If you also suffer from osteoarthritis, the choice to have surgery is more complicated. We'll talk more about this topic in the next section and in Chapter 9.

OSTEOARTHRITIS

Symptoms: Symptoms of osteoarthritis include knee pain, swelling, reduced knee flexibility, and knees that are stiffer in the morning or after activity. The actual process of osteoarthritis doesn't hurt. Your bones moving together without all of the stuffing or cushioning is the root of the pain.

Explanation: Osteoarthritis is known simply as "wear-and-tear arthritis." Also called *degenerative joint disease,* this arthritis affects the articular cartilage in our knees, the Teflon-like coating on the ends of the bones. If you picture this cartilage as a mattress, osteoarthritis means the stuffing is starting to come out. As osteoarthritis develops, small bone growths called *osteophytes* or *bone spurs* can develop. Eventually these can break off and float in the joint; these floating bone spurs are called *loose bodies.*

Causes: Osteoarthritis is very common. Although young people can suffer from it, osteoarthritis becomes more common as we age. Roughly 12.1 percent of Americans over the age of twenty-five suffer from this type of arthritis, and the percentages increase dramatically with age. Usually, osteoarthritis symptoms do not occur until the age of fifty. Risk factors include being overweight and/or having a job that puts stress on the knee joint through bending. Specific occupations that have a researched link to knee osteoarthritis are dock and shipyard workers, as well as carpenters.

It's important to note that you may have osteoarthritis—wear and tear

FEMALES AND THE ACL

For roughly the last decade, many researchers have focused their energy on the following fact, reported in a 2008 *New York Times* article titled "The Uneven Playing Field": "Female athletes rupture their ACLs at rates as high as five times that of males." This statistic reflects ACL rupture rates in sports such as soccer, basketball, and volleyball.

Researchers have uncovered at least four theories to explain this high incidence of ACL injuries in women:

- Females' hormonal fluctuations may be related to increased ACL tear rates. This research focuses on how hormones affect the ACL, but results have been conflicting, with no definitive findings.
- Females have wider pelvises than do men, leading to greater stress on the knee joint and its ligaments.
- The *intercondylar notch,* the space between the two condyles, or bony protrusions, at the end of the femur or thighbone, is smaller and more A-shaped in women, which can grind and weaken the ACL.
- Biomechanical or neuromuscular differences between women and men may lead to more ACL tears in women. Females control and move their bodies differently than do men.

Researcher and biomechanist Tim Hewett, professor and director at Cincinnati Children's Hospital Sports Medicine Biodynamics Center, thinks research findings give the most support to the biomechanical/neuromuscular theory. The other three theories may factor into the higher female incidence of ACL tears, but the only factor females can readily change is the biomechanical difference. "After undertaking neuromuscular training, females can go out on the field or court to play and show changes in their injury risk profiles. Several studies showed drops in ACL injury risk between 20 to 80 percent," says Hewett.

In ACL injury prevention programs, girls teach their bodies to move in ways that support their knees better. Exercises and training focus on:

- Increasing muscular strength and core stability. Players learn to use all muscles, including pelvic, abdominal, and hamstring muscles to execute moves, as opposed to relying on the quadriceps muscles and ligaments.
- Increasing muscular balance so both legs are strong and flexible, as opposed to having a dominant leg.
- Learning how to jump and land correctly. Women tend to lock their knees when they move, instead of bending their knees. Participants also practice stopping and cutting correctly.

You can find information on ACL injury prevention programs online. Locate the PEP (Prevent injury, Enhance Performance) Program, created by the Santa Monica ACL Prevention Project, and search for Dynamic Neuromuscular Analysis (DNA) Training on the Cincinnati Children's Hospital Medical Center's website (see "Resources," at the end of this book).

on cartilage happens to everyone eventually—but you may not be suffering symptoms for this particular ailment. You might have no knee pain at all, but your MRI will show arthritic cartilage. Alternatively, you might have knee pain and an MRI that shows osteoarthritis, but the pain might be coming from another problem entirely. A thorough physician will know to look for all possible causes of pain before making a diagnosis.

Your chances of having symptomatic osteoarthritis in your knees is most dependent on three variables:

- History of injury: previous knee traumas lead to a greater incidence of disease.
- Family history: if your relatives and ancestors had degenerative arthritis, chances are you will, too.
- Present level of activity: people who lead active, athletic lives tend to suffer more from osteoarthritis.

Keep in mind that all three risk factors apply, although sometimes one variable will override another. If you injure your left knee enough times on the football field, you'll probably suffer from the symptoms of osteoarthritis in that knee eventually. The risks are higher for competitive athletes than for recreational players.

Treatment: If you are suffering from knee pain that seems to indicate osteoarthritis, book an appointment with your doctor to confirm your diagnosis. The treatments for osteoarthritis are numerous. First, there are several ways you can protect your knee joints. If you are overweight, losing weight will alleviate pain and slow the wear and tear on your knees. Joint-bearing sports may cause pain. Try low-impact exercise options, including swimming, cycling, walking, Pilates, yoga, or using an elliptical trainer. Regular exercise, stretching, and strengthening exercises help your knees maintain their range of motion and lessen pain. Learn the best postural and movement habits through the Alexander Technique or the Feldenkrais Method. Even something as simple as avoiding stairs can be helpful. You can also change your diet to ease inflammation. All of these approaches are described in this book. Refer to the following chapters for more information: Chapter 4, "Stretch Your Body"; Chapter 5, "Finding a Movement Professional"; Chapter 6, "Practices for the Mind"; Chapter 7, "Bodyworks"; and Chapter 8, "Foods, Herbs, and Supplements."

Ice and heat can ease your pain and swelling. Follow the R.I.C.E. recommendations described in the box "R.I.C.E.: Knee Injury Self-Care" on page 37. Heat options include the application of heating pads, moist heating pads, or even a slightly damp hand towel warmed up in your microwave. Hot showers or baths may feel good. Over-the-counter Thermacare heat packs also can increase blood flow. These can alleviate hurt during long car rides or airplane trips, during athletic activities, or while sleeping. You can alternate ice and heat options.

Since osteoarthritis is a chronic condition, ask for your doctor's input on medications. Topical creams, OTC NSAIDs, and acetaminophen are all options. Your care provider can recommend prescription medications. If you take NSAIDs often, even OTC ones, regular blood screening is a good idea.

If you have severe osteoarthritis, your primary care physician can help you create a physical plan for dealing with your condition, recommend a doctor who specializes in arthritis issues, or refer you to a physical therapist. Physical therapy for osteoarthritis is really about moving the knee every day. The more you move your knee, the more nutrition your knee receives.

This helps prevent degenerative changes, which worsen osteoarthritis. Of course, it hurts to move an arthritic knee, but not moving it at all actually can make it hurt more. Chicago-based physical therapist Annie O'Connor, PT, OCS, Cert. MDT, corporate director of Musculoskeletal Practice at Rehabilitation Institute of Chicago, explains that osteoarthritis patients need to treat movement like a prescription. "Once a day won't suffice. You have to move the knee two to three times a day. It's like brushing your teeth," says O'Connor.

Working with a physical therapist, you will learn a daily exercise program that will maintain your knee joint's mobility. Your physical therapist will look at your gait and perhaps recommend orthotics to correct your alignment. A knee brace or a cane might take pressure off the joint. You will also work on strengthening the surrounding muscles, especially the hamstring and quadriceps muscles. To find ways to create your own stretching and exercise regimen, turn to Chapter 4 or visit the Arthritis Foundation online (see "Resources" at the end of this book).

For severe osteoarthritis, other pain relief options include cortisone injections and viscosupplementation. Surgery for this condition is a last resort, to be undergone after you have exhausted all of your other options for pain relief. For more information about medications, injections, viscosupplementation, and surgical options, see Chapter 9.

PATELLAR TENDONITIS & TENDINOSIS

Symptoms: Individuals with patellar tendonitis will often have pain, tenderness, and possibly swelling at the front of the kneecap. The pain often strikes during activities such as jumping, squatting, climbing stairs, or running.

Explanation: Tendonitis is the inflammation of tendons in and around your knee. Tendons are the fibrous bands that connect muscles to bones. Patellar tendonitis is the inflammation of the tendon that links the base of the patella to the shinbone. As you may recall, the patella lives within the patellar tendon. This spot on the knee is below where all the quadriceps muscles have become one tendon that encases the kneecap, meaning that a lot of force concentrates right at the bottom of the kneecap. Tendonitis can also occur in the other knee tendons, including the hamstrings and quadriceps tendons. If the pain occurs above the kneecap where the quadriceps tendon inserts, this is often called patellofemoral syndrome; see Patellofemoral (Kneecap) Pain section in chapter 1.

If tendonitis becomes chronic, meaning the tendonitis goes on for more than three months, the collagen in this tissue can start to break down. Now it has become a chronic condition called *tendinosis*.

Causes: Tendons are injured through overuse or an acute injury. Most people who suffer from tendonitis are athletes. Patellar tendonitis is often called "jumper's knee." People with this injury either have an acute episode during a sporting activity or simply hurt the patellar tendon through repetitive motions during athletics. Sports commonly associated with tendonitis and tendinosis include basketball, volleyball, running, tennis, and soccer. Being overweight and having tight leg muscles can result in patellar tendonitis. If your knee hurts and you keep ignoring this pain, you may be developing tendonitis or tendinosis.

Treatment: For patellar tendonitis, you need to rest the affected knee, abstaining from the activities and sports that cause your knee to hurt. To alleviate pain and symptoms, use the R.I.C.E. method of self-care (see the box "R.I.C.E.: Knee Injury Self-Care" on page 37). Take OTC NSAIDs for pain and swelling relief, or take acetaminophen to lessen pain. Try wearing a knee compressive sleeve, available at your local pharmacy, to ease swelling and support your knee joint. Participate in low-impact forms of exercise such as swimming and walking, as long as these activities don't hurt your knee. A movement therapy such as yoga, Pilates, or the Alexander Technique may help strengthen your knee and leg. Bodyworks such as acupuncture or massage therapy or a meditation practice may also alleviate your pain. Eliminating foods that promote inflammation can be helpful. All of these approaches are described in this book. Refer to the following chapters for more information: Chapter 4, "Stretch Your Body"; Chapter 5, "Finding a Movement Professional"; Chapter 6, "Practices for the Mind"; Chapter 7, "Bodyworks"; Chapter 8, "Foods, Herbs, and Supplements"; and Chapter 9, "Western Medical Interventions."

Visit your doctor or a sports medicine physician, as well. If you don't relieve your tendonitis, you soon may have a case of tendinosis. Your care provider can see if you need orthotics to correct your gait, and she might recommend wearing an infrapatellar strap or brace to ease the stress on your patellar tendon.

Your physician can also refer you to a physical therapist to help you strengthen the muscles and balance your body mechanics. Often a person is experiencing tendinosis in the knee by the time he visits a physical therapist. Treatment for tendinosis is similar to tendonitis. Try the therapies and remedies mentioned above. Healing from tendinosis can take a long time; tendons can take nine months to a year to recover fully. Exercises for both tendonitis and tendinosis strengthen the surrounding knee muscles and promote flexibility, although completing physical therapy exercises can be a painful process. Both tendonitis and tendinosis are often related to training issues, so a physical therapist will help you look at your exercise regimen. Did you train too hard and too fast? You can also learn McConnell taping to ease structural problems. Ultrasound therapy and massage can help with the healing process.

Rarely, tendinosis needs to be surgically treated. If all other treatments have failed and you have been in pain for more than six months, talk about patellar tendon debridement with your doctor. For more information about knee surgery, see Chapter 9.

ILIOTIBIAL BAND SYNDROME

Symptoms: The outside of your knee joint hurts, usually near the end of your femur or thighbone, or below the knee where the IT band attaches to the tibia. Usually you are in more pain when you are moving. The side of your hip may hurt.

Explanation: The iliotibial band, or IT band, is a sheath of connective tissue that extends from the pelvis, down the outside of the hip, and then ends just below your knee at your shinbone. This broad band has to go over some rough patches, including a bony bump on the outside of the knee at the end of the thighbone. Often this is where IT syndrome flares up. Basically, this syndrome is an irritation of the IT band.

Causes: IT band syndrome is caused by highly repetitive activities such as cycling, running, and hiking, especially on hilly terrain or on a banked surface such as the shoulder of a road. If you increase your mileage too quickly

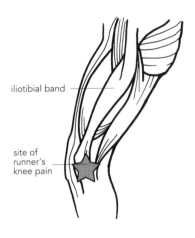

iliotibial band

site of
runner's
knee pain

2.4 Iliotibial Band

with any of these sports, IT band syndrome may result. Training issues such as exercising too much can also lead to iliotibial band syndrome. If you are bow-legged or have uneven leg length (excessive wear on the outside of your running shoe is a sign of these traits), you may be predisposed to this syndrome. Other sports associated with this injury include weight lifting and court sports such as racquetball, tennis, and handball. Bicycling with your feet "toed-in" at an extreme angle can do this, too. Pregnancy or the after-effects of pregnancy can also be risk factors.

Treatment: Use the self-care treatments described in the "R.I.C.E.: Knee Injury Self-Care" box on page 37. Limit excessive training. You can try using a foam roller on your IT band to loosen it, although sometimes this is too painful. To use this method, place a foam roller underneath your IT band and roll this section of your leg back and forth.

As outlined below, a variety of therapies and treatments are available for helping you deal with iliotibial band syndrome. These therapies are discussed in upcoming chapters of this book.

- Take OTC NSAIDs or acetaminophen for pain relief (remember that only NSAIDs help ease inflammation). See Chapter 9 to learn about such medications.

- Exercises and stretches that strengthen your IT band, your hip adductors, the buttocks, the core, and the pelvic floor muscles can help you avoid another IT band syndrome episode. Chapter 4 illustrates numerous exercises and stretches for your knee.
- Movement therapies such as Pilates, yoga, and the Feldenkrais Method can help you with postural issues that contribute to this injury and help strengthen your IT band and its surrounding muscles. Chapter 5 describes a number of helpful movement therapies.
- Practicing meditation can alleviate pain; see Chapter 6 for more information.
- Massage therapy or acupuncture may alleviate pain. See Chapter 7 for information about these and other bodyworks therapies.
- Making changes to your diet may ease inflammation; see Chapter 8 for more information.
- Orthotics might help correct alignment issues that are causing iliotibial pain. See the box in Chapter 1, "Keep Your Feet Happy."

Pay a visit to your doctor or a sports medicine physician as well. She can prescribe treatment with a physical therapist who can create an exercise regimen for you. Sometimes IT syndrome is related to your body architecture and alignment. This might mean it is impossible to do some activities, such as running, pain free. Your physical therapist can help explore this possibility with you. Sometimes, if other options fail, your doctor will try a cortisone injection. If the IT band does not respond to treatment, perhaps the actual problem is a lumbar spine issue; ask your doctor to investigate this possibility. Surgical intervention for IT syndrome is extremely rare.

LESS COMMON PROBLEMS

You can compromise the biggest joint in your body in many ways. The knee's mobility makes it an easier target than your other joints. The injuries listed above are the most common hurts that plague the average American's knee. People who compete in high-level athletics can harm their knees in less-obvious pain patterns. Other risk factors for knee problems include obesity; body structure abnormalities such as misaligned knees; weak muscle flexibility and strength; participation in repetitive activities including gardening, cycling, and running; or previous knee injuries. The following problems do not occur as often as the injuries we have already discussed.

STRAINS AND TEARS OF LCL AND PCL

It is rare for anyone other than a competitive athlete to strain or tear the LCL or PCL (lateral collateral ligament and posterior cruciate ligament). PCLs suffer disruptions during car accidents. It is unusual for the LCL ligament to tear without another ligament, such as the PCL, being injured as well. When more than one ligament tears, usually one or both of the ligaments need to be surgically repaired. If you tear your LCL or your PCL, physical rehabilitation leads to healing.

Bursitis

Bursitis is a commonly heard term. *Bursae* are the fluid-filled sacs around the knee that help cushion the joint. Bursitis means a bursa is inflamed or swollen. One type of knee bursitis is in the front of the kneecap; it is called *prepatellar bursitis* or *housemaid's knee.* Usually this type of bursitis occurs because of a repetitive work motion that creates sustained pressure on the knees, such as laying carpet, gardening, or scrubbing floors. Trauma can precede prepatellar bursitis as well, such as falling on your kneecap while playing soccer.

Pes anserine bursitis can result from sports that require side-to-side movement or cutting, such as basketball, soccer, or racquet sports. It also occurs in swimmers who specialize in the breaststroke and in middle-aged women who suffer from osteoarthritis. Being overweight can predispose you to this kind of bursitis. Usually people with pes anserine bursitis have pain and tenderness on the inside of the knee below their knee joint, especially when going up and down stairs. (Remember, this bursa is underneath the pes anserinus tendon, located a few centimeters below the knee joint.)

For any kind of bursitis, the treatment includes rest, ice, and anti-inflammatory medications. Bursitis requires medical attention because inflamed bursae may become infected. If your bursitis is not getting better, you may need either a cortisone shot or aspiration; see Chapter 9 for more information.

Tendon Rupture

A tendon rupture happens during a traumatic injury; such an event completely rips the tendon, possibly tearing it away from the attached bone. The patellar and quadriceps tendons are most likely to rupture. Although this injury is extraordinarily rare, it does require surgery.

Osgood-Schlatters and Sinding-Larsen-Johansson Diseases

Young athletes can suffer from Osgood-Schlatters disease or Sinding-Larsen-Johansson disease. Both of these overuse injuries occur if the individual's bones are still growing, affecting the growth plates at the ends of bone where growth is still happening. With Osgood-Schlatters disease, you can get swelling and tenderness on the bump on the shinbone just underneath the knee (the tibial tuberosity). With Sinding-Larsen-Johansson disease, you may get pain at the bottom edge of the kneecap. These conditions are usually diagnosed in boys between the ages of ten and fifteen, and in girls between the ages of eight and thirteen. Both injuries happen when the patellar tendon tugs on different parts of the tibia growth plates, causing pain and swelling. Super-athletic kids who participate in several sports are most likely to suffer from one of these conditions. Treatment involves modifying activities that cause pain, and stopping certain sports until individuals are skeletally mature.

Baker's Cysts

Baker's cysts can be caused by anything that causes joint swelling, such as osteoarthritis, traumatic knee injuries such as ligament or meniscal tears, and infections. The excess fluid in the joint bulges to the back of the knee and causes a Baker's cyst. Treat the injury that caused the cyst to form in the first place. In addition, you may need to use anti-inflammatory medications or see your doctor for a cortisone injection or to have the fluid removed.

Osteochrondritis Dissecans and Osteonecrosis

Osteochrondritis dissecans is another condition that affects younger people, this time adolescents and young adults, especially if they are active in sports. You may have pain and locking in your joints, especially with repetitive, impact sports that include a lot of jumping, such as basketball. Young adults with this syndrome who are not treated have a higher risk for developing osteoarthritis. A small area of bone and cartilage dies after the bone's blood supply is lost. Like a pothole in a slab of concrete, this dead bone can break off and float around. Treatment includes rest, anti-inflammatory medications, avoiding sports, and physical therapy. Sometimes you will need a brace or crutches. People may need surgery if they have symptoms for more than three months or if they are not getting better. *Osteonecrosis* means "bone death" and is a similar condition that usually affects just bone. This condition, though, usually happens in older adults. These floating pieces of bone or bone and cartilage are called *loose bodies* (like the loose bone spurs caused by osteoarthritis).

A Dislocated Kneecap or Patellar Disruption

A dislocated kneecap, or patellar disruption, is quite rare, happening to athletes participating in cutting sports. Like ACL tears, they occur when a foot stays planted but the leg keeps moving. People with certain anatomical tendencies can also dislocate their knees more often, and these injuries can happen off the sports court.

And the List Goes On...

Occasionally, pain on the medial side of the knee is actually referred pain from the hip. You can get a stress fracture in your patella. Gout, a metabolic disorder, can affect the knee; this is what people are referring to when they talk about "crystals" in the knee. You can also have autoimmune diseases that affect your knee, such as rheumatoid arthritis. Still, such conditions are less common, as are the knee problems not described in this book. In the following chapters, we will focus on explaining remedies for the most common knee ailments.

3 YOUR KNEES AND THE SPORTS YOU PLAY

OVER A LIFETIME, YOUR KNEES SEE A LOT OF ACTION. When you are young, your knees are not loud complainers. You run, you jump, and you literally bound up and down any set of stairs like Tigger in a *Winnie the Pooh* movie. Later, though, your knees creak and pop and you might feel some general achiness, especially during playtime.

We will all suffer some knee joint wear-and-tear as we age. If you are an avid competitor, an occasional runner, or a weekend hiker, it's time to pay attention to those lovely hinge joints. Protecting your knees while you play sports or engage in your favorite outdoor activities will pay off, preventing injury down the road.

In the following sections, we will look at various sports in relation to your knees. We've gathered insider tips and stretching suggestions for several athletic endeavors, as well as information on keeping your feet happy. (Seriously, your knees will thank you if your feet feel good.)

HIKING

Knee trouble often strikes hikers as they are walking downhill. Lean forward from your hips instead of walking upright as you descend an incline. This will help disperse the stress among your knees, hips, and ankles. For hikers, overall leg strength is important, and stretching those tight muscles after a hike is essential, too. If you practice yoga, the warrior pose is a good knee-strengthening asana (see Chapter 4). If you have an injured knee, however, avoid this pose. Climbing a lot of hills, especially with a load, can aggravate patellofemoral pain.

Use the same strategy as you hike uphill. Again, you should incline your body forward from the hips, says Seattle-area physical therapist Ellen Roth. If a hiker stays upright, especially when carrying a backpack, he is relying more on his hamstring muscles. Following the mountain's incline forces you to use your quadriceps and gluteus muscles as well.

If you hike on a regular basis, it is essential to buy hiking boots that fit you well. Purchase your footwear at an outdoor recreation or sporting goods store with staff members who understand how to fit you correctly. There are three kinds of hiking boots:

- Light hiking boots or hiking shoes. These are good for well-worn trails and hiking while wearing light day packs. Usually these shoes are made out of Gortex and they don't extend all the way up the ankle.
- Backpacking hiking boots. These boots are usually waterproof and they come up past the ankle, giving the hiker excellent ankle support for steeper inclines, muddy and slippery hikes, and uneven paths.
- Mountaineering boots. These hiking boots are much heavier than the other two options. They have a stiff shank, meaning you cannot bend the

boot easily. These are for serious hikers who carry heavy packs. Often these shoes are designed so the hiker can attach crampons to them for icy snow travel.

SKIING

As you ski downhill, your knee ligaments are already on stretch, keeping the femur from shearing over the tibia. ACL tears are common ski accidents. Skiers need to have strong leg muscles and flexibility; if you are a skier, consider working with a trainer to develop leg-strengthening regimes. Focusing on your balance during your off-the-slope workouts is also a good idea. At the gym, balance on a BOSU ball. Challenge your proprioception skills by closing your eyes while balancing. At home, work on balance and leg strength by using Wii Fit's balance board games or yoga program.

Make sure your ski boots fit. Have a ski mechanic service your ski bindings often. Some professionals recommend servicing your skis once a month or, at the very least, having them checked before ski season begins. Your local ski shop should also be following the American Society for Testing and Materials standard-release settings for alpine ski boots. The person adjusting your bindings or helping you select boots will want to know your age and body weight.

BIKING

Your local bike store's experts can help prevent knee injuries. Call and ask if you can get a bike fitting. A knowledgable staff member will have you sit on your bike and pedal, checking that the seat and handlebars are each in the right position for your body.

Wear cleats that clip right into your bike pedals. If your feet aren't clipped in, you may be relying on your quadriceps muscles for the majority of your pedal stroke, and your stroke will be choppy instead of a smooth circle. Clipping your shoes into your pedals forces you to use a wider range of leg muscles as you pedal, maintaining overall leg strength throughout the stroke. When you are biking, aim each knee toward the center of each side of your handlebars. As you pedal, be aware of your sits bones: they should be moving as little as possible.

Riding a single-speed or fixed-gear bike puts a lot of pressure on your knees, which can lead to stress and even injury. Spinning your wheels while riding alleviates knee pressure. Changing gears allows a rider to pedal and spin the bike's wheels as often as possible.

RUNNING

As you run, you want your body parts to absorb equally the shock of hitting the ground repetitively. If your form is off or your body isn't balanced strength-wise, one part may be absorbing all the shock: your foot arches, knees, hips, or your low back. Balance tight muscles—whether you feel tightness in your hips or buttocks muscles or someplace else—with flexibility. Take time every evening to stretch and lengthen your muscles.

Proper body mechanics can prevent injury. A running coach can watch you run, examining your body mechanics and spotting any abnormalities, from pronating feet to hunched shoulders. It is also a good idea to buy shoes at a shoe store geared toward runners. The shoe fitter can look at your current shoes' wear patterns and watch you run in a series of new shoes to see which model fits your body mechanics and foot best. The foot bed of your running shoe should feel comfortable. There should be plenty of room in the toe bed, meaning your toes shouldn't press too hard against the shoe. Your foot should not shift from front-to-back or side-to-side as you run. On the other hand, your feet shouldn't feel overly supported in the arch or too close to the sides of the shoe. Basically, your feet shouldn't feel too hemmed in by the shoe.

If you aren't familiar with any local running coaches, ask the clerks at your local running shoe store for names of coaches. Running coaches can help you design a training program as well as a stretching and strengthening regimen.

SOCCER

Soccer players tend to have a dominant leg that they usually use when kicking the ball. It's important to build strength in the other leg as well, balancing the body. The hip flexor and quadriceps muscles also tend to be the strongest muscles in a soccer player's legs. In the dominant leg the inside muscles may not be as strong as the outside muscles, leading to imbalance and injury. Strengthen those other leg muscles, too.

Often there isn't time during practice, before, or after games for strengthening the less-used muscles or even for stretching the most-used muscles. Stretch outside of practice and think about training with an exercise professional to create an individualized strength and flexibility plan. Cross-training by participating in other sports can help create body balance and overall strength.

GOLF, TENNIS, AND RACQUETBALL

Golf, tennis, or racquetball players usually focus on rotating specific areas of their bodies. Unfortunately, sometimes a player is rotating the wrong body section. During all these sports, you should be rotating your neck and upper back, hips, feet, and ankles. There should not be much rotation in your low back, sacroiliac joints, and knees. To stabilize the appropriate sections and mobilize the other areas, tighten and set your core muscles while practicing those golf or racquet swings. Focus on mobilizing the appropriate body sections while you practice. To slow down your movements, tie a piece of stretch band to your racquet or golf club; this makes it easier to practice correctly.

These sports tend to be one-sided, meaning you use the dominant, powerful side of your body for most of your moves. It's important to strengthen your less-dominant side as well, balancing your body.

BASKETBALL AND VOLLEYBALL

Both basketball and volleyball involve a lot of jumping and landing, as well as making quick changes of direction. Players of either sport can benefit from doing plyometric training exercises. Plyometrics are simply jumping exercises. These dynamic movements stretch the muscles and train the body for specific sports, helping improve your performance and prevent injury.

Although it's best to learn plyometrics from an exercise specialist, the most basic plyometric movement is jumping. Simply jumping rope can help you excel at jumping and landing during your favorite court sport. Leap side-to-side over a bamboo pole or bounce on a trampoline. Teach yourself to jump with good body posture by watching yourself in a mirror. Keep your feet straight and your thighs slightly rolled out. Take off and land in this position, keeping your knees from rolling in or rolling out excessively. You are looking for a straight line through your ankle, knee, and hip. Make sure to bend your knees as you jump and land.

4 STRETCH YOUR BODY

OUR BODIES WERE MADE TO MOVE. We are not sedentary creatures. Long ago, we did not spend all our time sitting by the fire. When we are injury-free, an all-day hike makes us feel more alive. Perhaps your Wednesday night soccer game is your favorite weekly event. Even though weeding your garden is a chore, there is some pleasure in tending to your vegetable plot every evening.

Participation in these activities is dependent on your pivotal hinge joints. Keeping your knees in good working order takes balance. The muscles supporting knee movement need to be strong yet flexible. "Any exercise shortens or tightens muscles. What's really important is to do as much stretching as you are exercising," says Laura Yon-Brook, MA, LMP, RYT, a sports medicine professional and yoga teacher who has worked with professional athletes. Stretching and lengthening those muscles will cause less pressure and wear and tear on the knee joint.

Some people don't find it difficult to spend time every day stretching their bodies, actually looking forward to the daily routine. Others list stretching as the last item on their to-do lists. The key to success might be making stretching more compelling. If you love your weekly yoga class, insert yoga poses into your list of exercises. Try various stretches until you have a selection of moves that you enjoy.

Spend time stretching in the evening after your muscles are warm from the day's activities. Try creating a routine from the stretches described in this chapter. For a program tailor-made for your body and the sports you participate in, work with a professional trained in exercise physiology. (See Chapter 5 to learn about various types of fitness professionals and how to select the best one for your situation.)

In this chapter, you'll find numerous exercises designed to keep your knees and their surrounding elements strong, balanced, and flexible. We'll also look at the way you move during your daily life, from how you sit while working on your computer, to the way you pick up your forty-pound backpack.

Important note: Use some of the gentler stretches as self-therapy for minor injuries. If you have a more serious knee injury, please work with a trained professional—a physical therapist, a sports medicine doctor, and/or a qualified instructor in yoga, the Alexander Technique, or any other practice described in subsequent chapters—before doing these stretches on your own. After your knee feels better, you can perform the stretches described below independently, with no danger of hurting yourself. See Chapter 5, "Finding a Movement Professional," for information about locating experts in these respective fields.

STRETCHING 1, 2, 3, 4

Four simple stretches can help promote proper knee movement.

Simple Stretch #1

The first move strengthens the deep hip lateral rotator muscles. When these muscles are weak, the tensor fascia lata (TFL), a muscle that starts in the pelvis and inserts into the iliotibial (IT) band, can dominate your movements. This domination can lead to knee problems.

1. Lie on your stomach and tighten your abdominal muscles.

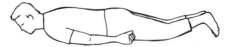

2. Bend your knees 90 degrees. Squeeze your heels together.

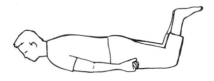

Simple Stretch #2

Sometimes the IT band rotates the tibia outward, which can contribute to knee pain. The second simple stretch rotates the tibia medially.

1. While sitting in a chair, cross your ankle over the knee of the opposite leg.
2. Grab onto your calf—with your thumbs on the inside of the calf and your fingers wrapped around the shinbone (tibia)—then rotate the shinbone upward. Your toes will move upward and your heel will move downward.

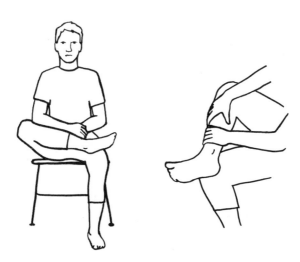

Simple Stretch #3

The third stretch strengthens the popliteus muscle, which sits behind the knee. Keeping this muscle strong helps keep the tibia from rotating excessively outward.

1. While sitting in a chair with your feet on the ground, use your lower leg muscles to move your leg inward.
2. Place your hand just below your knee to feel the tibia moving, keeping your knee still. Although your foot will move, make sure you are initiating the move with your tibia and not letting your knees come closer together.

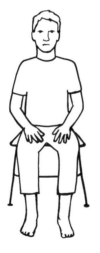 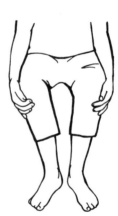

Simple Stretch #4

The fourth simple stretch involves the buttocks, or gluteal, muscles. When these muscles become tight, they can pull the leg outward, again negatively affecting the knee.

1. While sitting, cross your ankle over the knee of the opposite leg.
2. With your hands, pull your knee to your chest. You should feel your buttocks muscles stretching.

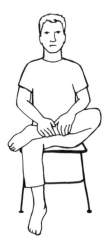
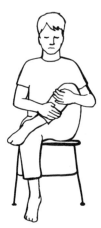

WORKSTATION 101

Many of us spend our workday at a computer station. Even if your work doesn't involve a computer, you may read the news online or spend a considerable amount of time surfing the Internet, emailing and instant messaging friends, or looking for new hiking locales and cheap flights for your next adventure. Sitting in a chair—even if a screen is not in front of you— is more stressful on your lower back than standing upright or lying down. What does this have to do with your knees? Often a knee injury stems from a back problem. Knee pain can be a direct result of poor sitting posture.

Have you ever heard the term *neutral posture*? This simply means you are in the most natural, relaxed position for your body. Think about how your body feels as you float in a lake—this is your neutral posture. When you are in this position, your body parts are well balanced, down to the right amount of space between your spinal column's vertebral bones. Using a well-designed chair can promote your best posture; ask your occupational or physical therapist for chair recommendations. Neutral Posture chairs, made by Neutral Posture, Inc., have won ergonomic awards (see "Resources" at the back of this book).

No matter what type of office chair you choose, using the following sitting and computer-work suggestions can prevent and ease strain on your low back and knees.

Sitting in a Chair
- Your hips should be slightly higher than your knees, or equal height to your knees. Pick the one that feels best to you.
- Your feet should be flat on the floor.

- If you are working at a computer, your chair back should be slightly re-clined, about 10 to 20 degrees, so you feel the space between your torso and your hips opening up a little bit.
- The chair back's curve should offer support at your lumbar or low spine. If not, add a rolled-up towel or a lumbar support pillow to support your natural back curve.

Working at a Computer

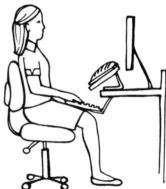

- Your elbows should be close to your body; this may mean not using the chair's armrests.
- Your hands should be level to your elbows, or a little below your elbows.
- Your wrists should be straight, with the forearms and hands in a straight line.
- You shouldn't have to reach too far for any item while working. Your mouse should be the same height as your keyboard and immediately next to your keyboard, within easy reach.
- Your shoulders should be relaxed. Sometimes using armrests can tighten up your shoulders.
- The computer screen should be eighteen to twenty-eight inches away, at eye-level or a little below eye-level.

If you find that sitting at a computer desk for hours strains your back, even though your body is in an ergonomically correct posture, try standing for part of your workday. You can stand while making phone calls—if you don't need to look at your monitor or type at the same time. You can also create a standing workstation. The ideal height for your keyboard and monitor depends on your height. Your computer screen should be at or just below eye-level. While you type, you should be able to maintain a comfortable body position with your shoulders relaxed. Make sure your elbows are bent between 70 to 90 degrees and keep your wrists straight.

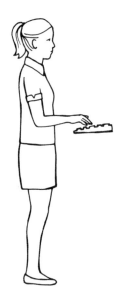

Another alternative to sitting in a chair is to use a fitness ball for short bursts of time. Sitting on a fitness ball helps build your core muscle tone and encourages you to vary your posture. However, sitting on a fitness ball is tiring, and it doesn't mean you will use your best posture. If you are not having an acute bout of back or knee pain, you can experiment with using a fitness ball. Perhaps super-fit competitive-level athletes can perch on fitness balls all day long, but most of us should work on a fitness ball for small "breaks" during office hours, adding up to roughly an hour or two.

Work Break Stretches

Good posture is also about varying movement. Seattle-area occupational therapist Carolyn Salazar, MS, tells her patients, "Your next posture is your best posture." Changing your position promotes blood flow and gets your muscles moving.

While this means making slight variations while you are standing or sitting, or getting up from sitting and taking a short walk once an hour, it's also vital to stretch throughout the workday. A study published in 2004 by the *European Journal of Applied Physiology and Occupational Physiology* found that "micropauses" can provide an immediate sense of relief and postpone the threshold for fatigue. A *micropause* is a short break of three to five seconds. Look away from the computer toward a spot in the distance and lift your hands off the keyboard to ease tension. Do this about every ten minutes. If stopping every ten minutes seems implausible, try taking a three- to five-minute stretch break once an hour. Micropauses can also ease eyestrain and prevent computer-related injury.

Often, moving your body in exactly the opposite way is helpful. If you are sitting in front of a computer, stand and do a backward bend. The lumbar rotation exercise can ease low-back stiffness.

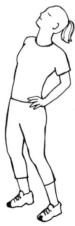

Backward Bend

1. Stand with your feet hip-distance apart. Place your hands on your hips.
2. Arch backward to make the hollow of your back deeper. Hold for three to five seconds.

Lumbar Rotation

1. While sitting, cross your arms and place each hand on its opposite shoulder.
2. Gently rotate your trunk from side to side in a small, pain-free range of motion.

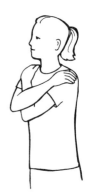

You can set a timer on your watch to remind yourself to take stretch breaks, or you can download various computer programs that will remind you to take periodic breaks. A popular program called "Stretch Break" has a computer-generated person perform stretches so you can simply follow along (turn to "Resources").

At the end of a long workday, or before going to sleep, stretch out your lower back again:

Knee-to-Chest Stretch

1. Lie on the floor on your back. Place your right hand behind your right knee.
2. Pull this knee in toward your chest until you feel a comfortable stretch in your lower back and buttocks. Keep your back relaxed.
3. Hold for five seconds. Repeat with your left knee.

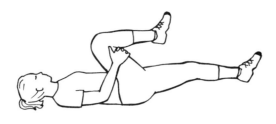

Lower Trunk Rotation Stretch

1. Lie on the floor with your back flat.
2. With your feet together, rotate your knees to the right side.
3. Hold for three to five seconds. Repeat, this time rotating your knees to the left side.

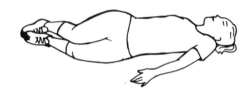

MOVE YOUR BODY EVERY DAY

Don't let knee pain stop you from being active—exercise is part of the cure. Of course, if you suffer from knee pain, you should check with your health-care provider before embarking on a new exercise regimen. Exercising on a regular basis is probably the most important activity you can do. Regular aerobic activity helps promote good posture and better sleep; increases the strength, endurance, and flexibility of muscles and other connective tissues; elevates your mood; decreases depression and anxiety; and helps manage stress.

It's ideal to move your body every day. Although you'll want to start off slowly and follow your doctor's guidelines, healthy adults under the age of sixty-five need thirty minutes of moderately intense physical exercise at

STRENGTH & FLEXIBILITY TRAINING

Maybe you have never been a gym rat. Perhaps you prefer exercising in the great outdoors or in the comfort of your home. If you don't visit a fitness club, there's a good chance you aren't lifting weights or doing resistance training. This type of work builds muscle mass and increases bone density. Strength training makes a body strong, aiding in the prevention of injury and helping the body deal more effectively with injury when it occurs. Ideally, a person should lift weights or work on resistance training for thirty minutes, two to three nonconsecutive days a week. A physical therapist, certified personal trainer, or a professional trained in exercise physiology can help you create a strength-training regimen.

least five times a week to stay in good health, according to recommendations released by the American College of Sports Medicine and the American Heart Association in 2007. How should you feel if you are working out at a moderate rate? You'll break a sweat and raise your heart rate, but you can still talk to your jogging partner.

If you sit at work all day, take walk breaks during office hours to counteract the effects of sitting. Before or after work, go for a swim, a bike ride, or a long walk. Even if you have a physical job, usually you are not engaged aerobically during your workday. To get that blood pumping, go for a run or schedule a squash game in the evening. If your job involves standing for the better part of eight hours, a bike ride or a swim will stretch and exercise your body in different ways. Even if you go kayaking or hiking every weekend, you need to fit in aerobic activities during the week.

Vary your aerobic activities for the best results. Swim one day, bicycle on another, run or speed-walk on another day. This cross-training will develop a variety of muscle groups and help muscles develop in a more complete way.

Feel too tired to exercise? Don't believe it. A University of Georgia study published in 2008 examined whether exercise could be used to treat fatigue. The fatigued participants engaged in either low- or high-intensity workouts three times a week for six weeks. At the end of the six weeks, they found that regular exercise had increased their energy levels by 20 percent. The study also found that the exercisers who participated in a low-intensity workout felt a 65 percent drop in tiredness, while the group doing more intense exercise felt only a 49 percent drop in fatigues. So taking an easy stroll after a long day might be even better than going for a long, intense run.

STRETCHES TO STRENGTHEN YOUR KNEES

Does stretching before a workout prevent injury? Results from studies on this question are inconclusive. However, a study published in 2005 in Norway showed that a pre-workout warm-up that included *dynamic* exercises did help prevent injuries.

What's the difference between static and dynamic stretches and exercises? Simple stretching is usually a static movement: you slowly move your body until you experience a mild pulling sensation, and then you hold the stretch for twenty to thirty seconds. Static stretches are probably best at the end of a workout (unless you are doing an exercise that requires a lot of flexibility, like gymnastics or ballet). Dynamic movement, on the other hand, means stretching the body while moving. In a dynamic warm-up, you move through a series of motions that you will use during your workout. This helps loosen muscles and tendons and increases the range of motion in various joints. Dynamic movement stretches can be helpful because they help warm up your muscles.

An aerobic warm-up, such as running for about five to ten minutes and then resting for five minutes before you work out, will literally warm you up, increasing blood circulation and body heat. An aerobic warm-up can also mean completing active pre-movement exercises.

If you are currently injury-free, American College of Sports Medicine (ACSM) personal trainer Sebastien Alary recommends completing a few of the following pre-movement exercises before your workouts. All of the following active stretches will help stretch and strengthen your knees and legs. Each stretch is described for one side of the body, but do each stretch bilaterally. For example, after your right leg is in the bent knee position, do the same stretch with your left knee bent. (If you never have practiced stretches similar to those described below, see Chapter 5, "Finding a Movement Professional," for information about finding a professional practitioner who can instruct you in how to perform these movement therapies.)

Resistance Band Knee Squat Exercise

1. Place a resistance band around both knees. Face forward, with your feet also facing forward and positioned slightly wider than hip-distance apart. Bend your knees. The tip of your knee will be just over your second toe.

2. With your elbows bent, walk forward, taking five steps. Stop and then walk backward to where you started. Keep pushing your knees out at all times and make sure to engage your buttocks muscles. Repeat three times.

3. Next, keep one leg planted and step forward and backward with the other leg. Keep pushing your knees out at all times and be sure to engage your buttocks muscles. Repeat ten times.

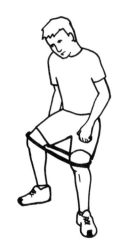

Resistance Band Leg Exercises

1. Attach one end of a resistance band to a stable piece of furniture or trap the end of the band in a closed door. (Place the end of the resistance band near the bottom of an open door and then quickly close the door, trapping the band in the shut doorway). Place your right leg in the other end of the resistance band, with the band at ankle level.

2. Face the piece of furniture or closed door, with your knees slightly bent and your elbows bent.

3. Slightly lift the leg in the resistance band. Initiate the leg movement with your hip and buttocks muscles, keeping your core

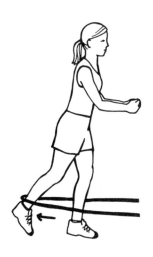

engaged and upper trunk as still as possible. Slowly move the leg backward and then forward. Do this five to ten times with each leg.

4. Now face away from the piece of furniture or closed door with the right leg again in the resistance band at ankle level.

5. Bend your left knee, so the knee is directly over your foot. Position your right leg behind your left, so you are in a lunge position.

6. With your elbows bent, move your right leg forward, bending the knee as you move and ending in a bent knee position. Then move your right leg backward until it is again in a lunge position. Remember to initiate the leg movement with your hip and buttocks muscles, keeping your core engaged and upper trunk as still as possible. Do this five to ten times with each leg.

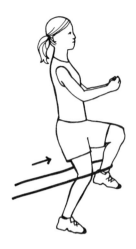

Resistance Band BOSU Ball Squat Exercise

1. Place a BOSU ball with the rounded half on the floor, so you can stand on the flat side. Place a resistance band around both legs, just above your knees.

2. Stand on the BOSU ball with your knees bent and your feet facing forward. Balance on the ball for as long as possible.

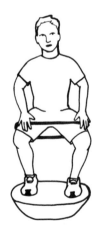

Resistance Band Squat Knee Straighten Exercise

1. You will need a partner for this exercise. Have your partner grasp one end of a resistance band, holding steady while you hold the other end.
2. Bend your elbows and both knees, so you look like you are sitting in a chair.
3. With your toes pointing up, slowly move your left foot forward, straightening your left leg. Keep your foot off the floor. When your leg is stretched out completely, slowly place your foot back on the floor again and bring your leg back into the bent knee position. Do this five to ten times with each leg.

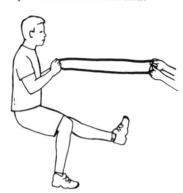

ACL TEAR PREVENTION MOVES

In Chapter 2, "Common Knee Problems," we discussed the high rate of ACL injuries in girls and women. Luckily, entire exercise and training programs exist to help prevent female ACL injuries (see "Resources," at the back of the book). The exercises below are from Cincinnati Children's Hospital Sports Medicine Biodynamics Center. These exercises were used in a study that analyzed neuromuscular training for preventing ACL injuries in female athletes. Originally designed for high school and college age female athletes, these exercises can also be beneficial to adult women and men. (Men tear their ACLs too!) Do these exercises two or three days a week or before your sports practice or competitions.

Lateral Jump and Hold

1. For the lateral jump and hold, stand with your feet close together and with your knees slightly bent.
2. Jump laterally over a line, keeping your knees bent and staying close to the line. When you land on the opposite side, descend into a deep knee bend and hold for five seconds. Do this four times.

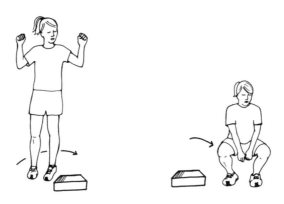

Lateral Hop and Hold

1. For the lateral hop and hold, stand on one foot with your knee slightly bent.
2. Jump sideways over a line, keeping your knee bent and staying close to the line. When you land on the opposite side, descend immediately into a single-leg deep knee bend and hold for five seconds. Do this six times, three times for each leg.

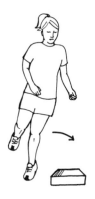
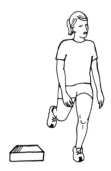

Front Lunges

1. Start in a standing position, with your feet about hip-distance apart.
2. Take one long step forward. The step should be exaggerated in length to the point that your front leg is positioned with the knee flexed to a 90-degree angle and the lower leg is completely vertical. The back leg should be as straight as possible and the torso upright. Get your hips as low as possible while maintaining this body position.
3. Drive off the front leg, pushing back to return to the original position. Do this exercise six times, starting the lunge on either side of your body three times.

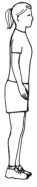
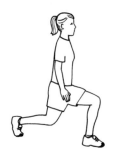

Walking Lunges

1. Perform the front lunge, but instead of returning to the start position, step through with the back leg and lunge forward with it.

2. Lunge each front leg far enough ahead that your knee does not advance beyond your ankle. Roll through a series of six to ten lunges.

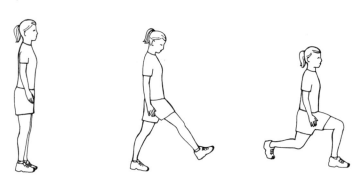

BOSU Pelvic Bridge

1. Lie face up on the floor or a mat with your hips in a vertical position, your knees bent, and your feet planted on the flat side of a BOSU ball. Tighten your core and buttocks muscles.

2. Lift your hips and trunk off the ground to execute a pelvic bridge. Hold this position for three seconds. Do this two times.

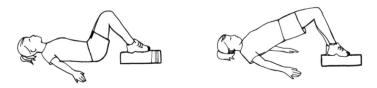

BOSU Single-Leg Pelvic Bridge

1. Lie face up on the floor or a mat with one hip in a vertical position, the knee bent, and the foot planted on the flat side of the BOSU. Fully extend the other leg. Tighten your core and buttocks muscles.
2. Lift your hips and elevate your trunk off the ground to execute a pelvic bridge.
1. Hold this position three seconds. Do this exercise twice with each leg.

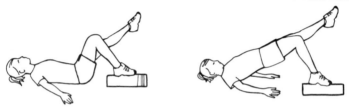

BOSU Toe Touch Swimmers

1. Begin in a prone position with your abdomen centered on the round side of a BOSU. Stretch yourself into a flying "Superman" pose, with your arms extended out in front of you and your legs stretched out behind.
2. Tighten your core and buttocks muscles.
3. Reach back with your right arm and bend your left leg. Touch your left foot and then return to the outstretched Superman position.
2. Do this ten times, using each arm and leg five times.

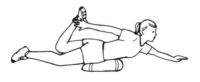
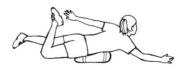

Prone Bridge Hip Extension Opposed Shoulder Flexion

1. Begin facedown with your elbows bent and balanced on an Airex pad and your legs straight out behind you with your toes on the ground.
2. Elevate the opposite arm and leg, holding this position for a single count.
3. Return to the start position. Do this ten times, five times for each side of the body.

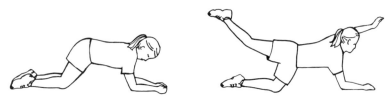

STRETCHES FOR PREVENTING KNEE PAIN

After a workout, your muscles are warmed up and capable of greater movement with less effort. By performing static stretches after your workout, you can more effectively lengthen a group of muscles, making muscles and connective tissues more flexible and less injury-prone. Muscles, tendons, ligaments, and joints that have a greater range of motion are not as likely to strain or tear.

Physical therapist Wolfgang Brolley recommends the following stretches for preventing knee injuries. Each stretch is described for one side of the body, but do each stretch bilaterally. For example, after doing a stretch with your right leg in the bent knee position, do the stretch with your left knee bent.

Hip Flexor Stretch

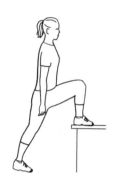

1. Put one foot up on a counter or other solid edge that is about the height of your hips.
2. Stand with a neutral spine* and with your other foot slightly behind you.
3. Tilt your pelvis and then push your hips toward the counter while holding neutral spine (see page 92).

Hip Adductor Stretch

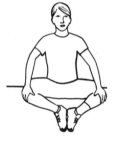

1. Sit with your back against a wall, your knees bent at a right angle, and the arches of your feet to-gether.
2. Maintain a neutral spine while using your hands to push gently down on your knees.
3. Hold for five to ten breaths.

Hamstring Stretch 1

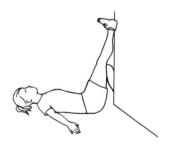

1. Lie on your back on the floor. Raise one leg and lean it up against a doorway. The opposite leg should be bent with the foot on the floor.
2. Straighten the leg leaning against the doorway and move your rear closer to the doorway to increase the stretch.

Hamstring Stretch 2

1. Lying on your back, clasp both hands behind one bent leg and straighten the other leg onto the floor.
2. Pull gently on your bent leg while slowly straightening your knee. (It's not necessary to straighten the knee and leg fully.) You should feel a gentle stretch.

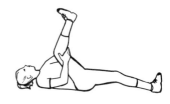

Heelcord Stretch 1

1. Face a wall with your feet staggered one in front of the other. Your rear foot should be pointing straight ahead and your rear knee should be straight.
2. Push your trunk toward the wall, maintaining the placement of your feet.

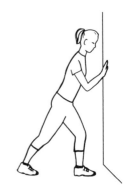

Heelcord Stretch 2

1. While wearing shoes, stand with the balls of your feet on the edge of a step.
2. Allow one heel to drop toward the ground while maintaining proper foot alignment.

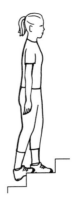

Quadriceps Stretch 1

1. Lie on your stomach with your belly button centered on a pillow.
2. Bend one knee, grasp the ankle with your hand (or use a belt), and pull your heel toward your buttocks.

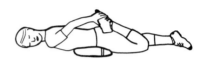

Quadriceps Stretch 2

1. Hook the top of your foot behind you on a desk.
2. Keeping neutral spine,* bend your opposite knee.
3. For a higher level of stretch, keep the knee of the stretched leg behind your hip.

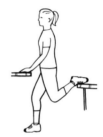

Iliotibial Band/Piriformis Stretch 1

1. While lying on your back, bend your right leg. Put your right hand behind your right knee and hold your right ankle with your left hand.
2. While maintaining neutral spine,* push your knee toward your opposite shoulder while pulling your ankle toward you.

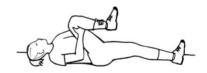

Iliotibial Band/Piriformis Stretch 2

1. Stand on one leg, with your right leg bent at the knee at a 90 degree angle (your knee will be directly in front of your hip); rest your bent leg on a hip-height surface.

2. You will feel a stretch in your right piriformis muscle. If your knee is lying flat on the table and you want to feel a deeper stretch, lean forward from your hips while maintaining a neutral spine.*

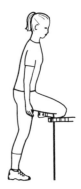

Neutral spine means your spine is essentially in a position that feels natural and comfortable to you. A physical therapist or exercise specialist can help you find this position. Alternatively, while standing, move your backbone and tilt your pelvis in various positions, seeing what feels best.

YOGA FOR YOUR KNEES

Yoga poses can stretch and strengthen your knees and legs. If you have knee issues, get your doctor's approval before starting a yoga practice. Yoga is not meant to replace medical care, but is instead an adjunct therapy. If you are new to yoga, it's best to learn with a certified instructor, either in a one-on–one setting or in a beginner's class.

Below are gentle postures (called *asanas*) that will stretch and strengthen the muscles around the knee and keep your knee joint healthy.

Goddess Pose

1. Stand with your feet apart, wider than the hips and feet facing forward. Turn your toes out slightly for balance.
2. Bend your knees to bring your torso down toward the floor. With your hands facing each other, bring your arms to a bent position at about 90 degree angles.
3. Lift your toes briefly to make sure your body is balanced and all your leg muscles are engaged, and then place your toes back on the floor.
4. Hold the pose for six to twelve breaths, breathing deeply in and out.

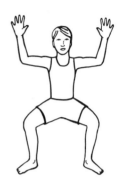

Warrior 2 Pose

1. Stand with your feet apart, wider than the hips, with feet facing forward.
2. Turn your right foot so it points outward.
3. As you engage your core and pelvic muscles, bend your right knee, bringing the knee directly above the right foot.
4. Lift your arms straight out to your sides with palms facing down.
5. Turn your head to face your extended right arm. Make sure your shoulders are relaxed, dropping them away from your ears.
6. Hold the pose for six to twelve breaths, breathing deeply in and out. Switch sides.

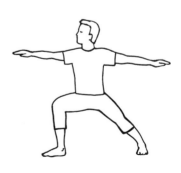

Wide-Legged Forward Bend

1. Stand with your feet apart, wider than the hips, with feet facing forward.
2. As you engage the core and pelvic muscles, bend forward from the hips, placing your palms on the ground. If you cannot touch the floor, place your hands on a block, bending until you feel a gentle stretch.
3. Hold the pose for six to twelve breaths, breathing deeply in and out.

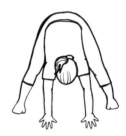

STAND UP STRAIGHT!

Can you hear your mom's voice in your head, reminding you not to slouch? She had your best interests in mind. Poor posture is one of the top contenders for causes of musculoskeletal disorders. Good posture means your body parts are in balance: the gentle S-curve of the spine is not overly exaggerated, and your muscles are strong and flexible, especially the abdomen, hip, and leg muscles. From a side view, an imaginary line should run down through your ear, shoulder, hip, knee, and ankle.

You can check your posture at home. Evaluate your standing posture with these tests from the American Physical Therapy Association.

To check for normal curves of the spine:

- Stand with your back to a wall, heels about three inches from the wall.

- Place one hand behind your neck, with the back of the hand against the wall, and the other hand behind your low back with the palm against the wall.

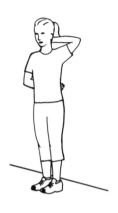

If there is excessive space between your back and the wall, such that you can easily move your hands forward and back more than one inch, some adjustment in your posture may be necessary to restore the normal curves of your spine.

  To check your posture from a front view, stand directly in front of a full-length mirror and answer the following questions:

- Is your head held straight (good posture) or does your held tilt to one side or another (bad posture)?
- Are your shoulders level (good posture) or is one shoulder lower than the other (bad posture)?
- Are the spaces between your sides and arms equal (good posture) or are the sides unequal (bad posture)?
- Are your hips level (good posture) or is one hip higher than the other (bad posture)?
- Do your kneecaps face straight ahead (good posture) or do either of your knees turn in or out (bad posture)?
- Are your ankles straight (good posture) or do your ankles roll in so that the weight is on the inside of your feet (bad posture)?

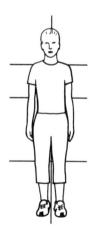

If you find your posture lacking, this could be contributing to your knee pain. Your primary care doctor can also evaluate your posture, or she might send you to a physical therapist for further review. Through physical therapy treatment, postural issues can be corrected by building muscle strength and flexibility and learning the best way for your body to stand, sit, and walk. You can also learn better postural traits through movement therapies, including the Feldenkrais Method, the Alexander Technique, Pilates, tai chi, and yoga.

5   FINDING A MOVEMENT PROFESSIONAL

SOMETIMES YOU CAN MANAGE KNEE PAIN without the help of professionals. Perhaps your knee is out-of-whack after a long marathon-training run. You take ibuprofen, ice your knee every four hours, spend extra time stretching, and watch how you move. After a few days of self-care, your pain has dissipated.

Other bouts of knee pain can leave you wondering who to call for help. Perhaps your right knee is extremely sore and painful after every soccer match, hurting for two days. This might be easy to ignore after a few games, but six months of consistent pain gets your attention. Perhaps you look forward to hiking every summer weekend, but this season you have canceled your next few outings thanks to the knee pain you experienced during your last mountain descent.

What type of health-care practitioner can ease your hurt and help start you on the road to healing? It may be as simple as learning a movement therapy such as yoga, Pilates, or Feldenkrais. If this doesn't help, it may be time to call a knee specialist.

After you suffer an acute knee injury, you need to strengthen your body in a specific way to prevent the injury from reoccurring. If you need knee surgery, physical therapy is usually a post-operative necessity. You may also seek professional help to learn how to deal with a chronic knee condition such as osteoarthritis.

YOGA

Moving your body is often the best thing you can do for yourself if you have minor knee pain. While this can mean moving your body through its daily routines, it also means exercising. If your knee pain has stopped you from practicing yoga, unroll your mat. A knowledgeable yoga teacher can adapt exercises to make them safe for your injured knee. This movement therapy can also help correct postural issues and muscular imbalances that led to your knee pain. It's not uncommon to hear stories of people with knee issues who found relief from practicing yoga.

If you have torn a ligament and are awaiting surgery, this isn't the time to start a yoga practice. After post-surgical rehabilitation, though, a yoga practice can help strengthen your joint and its surrounding muscles, preventing further injuries. If you are recovering from an acute knee injury, a yoga practice can be a good therapeutic movement practice. Ask your doctor or physical therapist if this is true for your particular case.

If you've never tried yoga, finding a place to start your practice shouldn't be a problem. Although yoga originated in India, where people have been practicing it for centuries, it has also become a familiar part of our exercise culture in America. You are likely to find a yoga program at your local health club, in a nearby hospital or health center, at your community center, or in a neighbor's basement studio.

Perhaps you think yoga is only for flexible people. "Saying 'I can't do yoga because I'm not flexible' is like saying 'I can't take guitar lessons because I don't know how to play guitar,'" says Valerie Crosby, a certified yoga teacher in Albuquerque, New Mexico.

Yoga is about intentional movement. "It's the practice of moving the body with the breath," explains Cathy Prescott, a senior teacher and mentor for Integrative Yoga Therapy who lives in Niskayuna, New York. "I talk with my hands, but this is not yoga. If I stop, take a breath, lift my arms, and exhale, that is yoga. I have to concentrate, breathe, and pay attention to the movement I make."

In India and the United States, developing self-understanding has always been one of the main principles of yoga. This self-understanding and unity is gained through yoga *poses* (also called *postures* or *asanas*), and breathing (called *pranayama*). Sometimes yoga includes meditation (*dhyana*). While practicing yoga, you will move into various postures and use various breathing techniques. Doing this stretches and strengthens your body and relaxes your mind. Intentional movement and breathing makes you aware of your body and helps place you in the present moment.

Yoga does not replace medical care; it is, instead, an adjunct treatment. Before you begin a yoga practice, check with your primary care physician to see if she feels you are ready to participate in yoga.

The Proof Is in the Practice

Yoga is good preventative medicine. Practicing yoga will make you more aware of how you move your body. You can carry this new awareness over into your athletic and recreational activities, learning to move in ways less likely to cause injury. For example, jumping with locked knees can be the precursor for an ACL injury. If a person knows this and is learning how to jump safely, a yoga practice can help her become more aware of her body movements. First, she thinks about how her body moves during yoga, and then she carries this awareness over into her movements on the athletic court.

Yoga also can help correct postural traits that cause knee pain. During a class, you always do poses with both sides of your body, helping to keep your body balanced. A yoga instructor versed in therapeutic practices will know how to design a practice for a person who is bowlegged, or knock-kneed, or someone with hyperextension issues or postural misalignment. This in turn can help protect your knees from injuries, since body alignment can be a risk factor for ACL tears in females, as well as knee injuries in either sex. Any part of the lower body—the ankle, knee, hip, or low back—can be misaligned or can move in a way that will eventually harm the knee. Yoga can help you bring your body back into alignment.

A muscular imbalance can also lead to knee pain. Perhaps the outer quadriceps muscle is stronger than the inner quadriceps muscle. Your abdominal muscles may be weak, causing you to put more pressure on your knee joint. Yoga strengthens muscles, leading to better muscle balance.

Yoga can also be a therapeutic practice for someone with osteoarthritis. "If you stop moving the [knee] joint, you will develop further problems," says yoga teacher Cathy Prescott. She adds that osteoarthritis patients can benefit from gentle motions that move the joint while the person isn't in a weight-bearing position.

How Yoga Helps Your Knees

The book *Yoga as Medicine,* by Timothy McCall, MD, describes forty specific ways a yoga practice can improve someone's health. Some of the reasons that point directly to improving knee function are that yoga:

- Improves balance
- Increases flexibility
- Strengthens muscles
- Improves posture
- Improves joint health
- Releases unconscious muscle gripping
- Relieves pain
- Reduces weight
- Increases oxygen supply to the tissues

Yoga can also improve a person's psychological health. Practicing yoga can reduce levels of stress hormones, lessen depression, and relax the nervous system. Of course, all of these healing benefits are intertwined. During yoga sessions, you'll breathe more slowly and deeply, which in turn will lead to a relaxation response in your body. An hour or more spent doing yoga also takes you out of your life and its immediate stresses, which can lift your mood and relax your body.

Yoga works to bring the body, mind, and spirit into balance, and some believe this is why yoga can promote healing in the body. During yoga practice, you are asked to be in the present moment, focusing on what is going on in both your body and mind. "We frequently neglect our bodies but we really can't separate out our thinking life from our physical life," says Jennifer Keeler, a certified yoga teacher who runs Yoga Momma at the

Phinney Yoga House in Seattle. "Yoga brings our whole self into connection again. It allows us to recognize when we are stressed and out of balance, how the stress is affecting our overall well-being. Then it provides tools to begin making changes in our actions resulting in balance."

Yoga also helps people take charge of their own health care. The more you learn about how your body feels and how your mind works, the more you can figure out what therapies are best for your own medical issues.

Types of Yoga

If you suffer from knee pain or have had knee surgery, choose a yoga style with care. There are numerous types of yoga, and some are more appropriate than others are for people with knee issues. People with frequent knee pain should avoid:

- Ashtanga, or Power, yoga
- Bikram, or Hot, yoga
- Vinyasa yoga
- Some yoga classes at a gym

The above yoga styles focus on more vigorous movement: participants move quickly between poses, without time to make adaptations for knee issues. Some gym classes might be appropriate for people with knee problems; look for gentle yoga classes or therapeutic classes.

Yoga styles that are more appropriate for individuals with knee concerns include:

- Iyengar yoga
- Viniyoga yoga

- Kripalu yoga
- Phoenix Rising Yoga Therapy
- Anusara yoga
- Integral yoga

Often a studio is not aligned with one specific yoga style. Teachers may have studied several types of yoga. The name a teacher gives her studio is often a synthesis of all she has learned during various trainings and through years of teaching yoga.

If, during your search, you come across a yoga style you don't recognize, ask the instructor if this style is appropriate for your knee issue. You should be able to adapt poses to fit your body's needs and minimize the risk of injury, and the teachers should have experience working with people with knee problems.

Finding a Yoga Instructor

Finding the right yoga teacher is as important as choosing an appropriate style of yoga. If you have knee issues, look for a studio with gentle or beginner-level classes. Some practitioners obtain a Yoga Alliance Membership (see "Resources," at the end of this book). This national organization helps lead the yoga movement in the United States by setting standards, fostering integrity, providing resources, and upholding the teachings of yoga. Refer to their website for information about finding an instructor.

Make sure your yoga instructor is trained and certified. There are no federal regulations in place, but there may be local regulations in your state. Whatever yoga style a teacher trains in, she should have completed at least a 200-hour level of training. Often instructors have completed training in

YOGIC BREATHING

You can use the breathing practices you learn in a yoga class in your daily life. You can change your mood with your breath. Try this exercise: first, think about how you feel at this moment. Now take five deep breaths in a row, while focusing on your breath. How do you feel now?

Our breathing becomes shallow and short when we are nervous or in pain. Simply by stopping and breathing deeply, we can influence our emotions, lessen fear and pain, and relieve stress.

Yogic breathing, also called diaphragmatic breathing, is a simple relaxation exercise that anyone can learn:

- Put your hands on your stomach. Imagine that your belly is an inflatable mattress.
- Blow all your air out while imagining that the mattress is deflating. Your belly will shrink in.
- Take a deep breath in and feel the mattress—your belly—inflate.

Most people breathe only from their chest up. Yogic breathing forces people to take deeper breaths, so they relax more effectively. One of the simplest, easiest ways to relax is to do ten of these breaths in a row.

more than one style; this diversity and depth of knowledge can be beneficial to students.

Call or meet with a potential yoga teacher. Ask the teacher the following questions:

- What kind of experience do you have working with people with knee pain?
- Do you know how to adapt poses for someone with knee issues?
- What yoga training have you done?

If the teacher has never worked with people with knee problems, she might not be the right instructor for you. You should feel comfortable with the teacher, since you will want to talk with her about adapting a pose when it doesn't feel right, or chat before class if you are having a flare-up of pain.

The potential teacher should also ask you what you want out of a yoga class. The studio should have a variety of classes, and asking this question will help the teacher determine what class is the best fit for you. Before you pick a yoga class, think about what you hope to gain from your practice. Some classes or teachers will be more appropriate than others for your needs. Are you looking for quiet, reflective time? Do you want a class that includes meditation or chanting? Are you hoping yoga will help you de-stress and relax? Everyone is unique, but the instructor can help create a practice that works for you.

Your yoga teacher should be able to meet you where you are, physically and mentally. This means that if you are suffering from knee pain or re-cently had surgery, it's a good idea to have a few individual sessions—just you and the teacher—before joining a class. Tell the instructor about your doctor's diagnosis, your symptoms, and how you feel as you hold yoga pos-tures. The teacher can observe how your body is moving, help you modify poses, and determine what class is appropriate for you. Perhaps you need to practice yoga while sitting, or use blocks and straps for some poses, or avoid some moves altogether. When you do join a class, the instructor will be able to tell you what poses to avoid and adaptations you need to make to other poses during class. More importantly, you'll know more about yoga and what moves and modifications are appropriate for you. You will learn what is best for your body.

Yoga Class

Remember that during a yoga class what is happening on your mat is the most important aspect of your session. Perhaps some students seem more flexible than you, or another person's pose looks different from yours. The point of yoga is not about being super flexible or holding a posture so it looks like the one portrayed in a book. "It doesn't matter how you look, it matters how you feel. Can you breathe in the pose, and what happens in your mind?" asks Cathy Prescott, a yoga teacher based in Niskayuna, New York. "The postures are about finding a balance between effort and ease. You should be working just enough and relaxed just enough."

Protect your knees from further injury while practicing yoga. Always talk with an instructor about your specific knee concerns. Below is a list of adaptations that instructors often recommend for people who are either currently suffering from knee pain or have had knee injuries in the past:

- The knee should always be directly above the ankle. If you are in a bent knee position, such as a lunge, make sure the knee is directly in line with the ankle.
- If your bent knee is on the mat, place a folded blanket or some type of soft padding under the knee.
- It's important to balance your body's weight with proper foot alignment. To make sure the weight is being distributed evenly, lift up your toes for a moment.

- Sometimes people with knee pain shouldn't keep their legs straight during poses. Working with your knees slightly bent will also stretch and strengthen your body.

When you do a yoga pose, you should feel a stretch and be able to breathe. Stop and move out of a posture if you feel pain beyond the normal feeling of a muscle stretch. If you experience any grinding motion, heat, or sharp pains, this is also your cue to stop and talk to the teacher. This pose may not be appropriate for your body, or you may need to adapt the pose by using props, or by moving your body in a different way.

Setting Up a Home Yoga Practice

While taking a yoga class even just once a week is beneficial, practicing yoga more often is better. Although a group class can create community and people can challenge one another in class, a daily home practice will reap the most benefits for someone with knee issues. If you suffer from osteoarthritis, moving your knee every day is important. For an osteoarthritis patient, as well as any person experiencing knee pain, it is vital to work with a yoga teacher who is versed in therapeutic yoga as you set up a home practice.

If you are taking private classes with an instructor, she can help you set up a home practice. If you are currently in a group class, it's easiest to set up a home practice by having a one-on-one session with your teacher. Teacher Cathy Prescott likes to help her students create three distinct practices, each fifteen to twenty minutes in length. These short sessions can be put together if a person feels like doing a longer session on a particular day.

Meeting with a teacher helps you learn the poses correctly and helps you figure out what props you will need to use at home. Starting a home practice often means investing in yoga equipment including blocks, straps, bolsters, or stools. Sometimes, using a chair or pillow you already own will suffice, and a wall is often an excellent prop.

An instructor might recommend just two to three yoga postures to do every day. Doing each pose correctly, with attention focused on your body and mind, is often the most vital part of practice. When you are ready to change your daily practice, meet with your instructor again. Fort some that is after a month, while other people find changing their home practice every six months works for them.

PILATES

Pilates isn't an ancient art, but its origin story is compelling. Joseph Pilates, born in Germany in 1880, created his own fitness regimen to help himself overcome several childhood illnesses. He believed his mind led his body to healing, and that others could follow a similar path through his fitness regimen. While held as a prisoner during World War I, he taught exercises to the other prisoners. He leaned the prison beds' box springs against the wall and attached slings to them. The prisoners did various stretches with the help of the beds and slings, which were the very first Pilates exercise machines.

In the late 1920s, Joseph Pilates immigrated to the United States. Along with his wife, Clara, he started an exercise gym in New York City. Many of his first devotees were professional dancers. Today dancers worldwide use his methods to stay in shape and help recover from injury. After Pilates died in 1967, people continued to teach his basic mind/body fitness regimen, and this became known as the Pilates Method.

TAI CHI

If you go to any park in China or Southeast Asia, chances are you will see hundreds of people of all ages practicing the graceful dance-like movements of *tai chi*. Also known as *tai qi* or *tai chi chu'an*, this ancient art form has been practiced in China for thousands of years. Tai chi is both a martial art and a health-promoting mind–body exercise regimen. The hundreds of movements that comprise this practice lessen stress by encouraging deep, slow breathing; improving flexibility and circulation; and building strength in the lower legs and hips. Tai chi can also be used as an adjunct therapy for people suffering from knee pain. Practicing tai chi on a regular basis can improve body alignment, helping your knee movements become more supple and fluent, which can lessen your pain.

There are many tai chi styles. Some are practiced quite slowly while others forms have participants moving fast and vigorously. To pick a class that fits your needs, observe or try a few different types of classes.

Quality of Movement

Today's Pilates practices have evolved from Joseph's original teachings. Well-trained teachers combine new knowledge about anatomy and movement, making current exercises more beneficial for students. Pilates is an exercise system that emphasizes breathing, concentration, control, precision, centering, and flow. With this focus, students work on spinal and pelvic alignment and core strength while performing exercises.

Although it's a heady proposition to keep six attributes in mind while executing exercises, this simply means that Pilates is about being conscious about your movements. These are tools used to create precise movements. "Pilates is about quality of movement more than the quantity of repetitions. Beautifully executing three sets of an exercise with control, precision, and proper breathing is much more beneficial than executing fifty repetitions without that focus to detail," says Marjorie Thompson, lead instructor and program director of the Pacific Northwest Ballet's Pilates program, PNB-Conditioning. "Breathing properly is essential to executing exercises efficiently. This carries over in your day-to-day life."

How Pilates Helps Your Knees

An acute knee injury or a chronic knee problem can stem from muscular imbalances. Although no one has perfect posture, postural alignment can play a role in knee pain as well. Pilates helps promote muscular balance by developing a person's core strength. Joseph's definition of the body's "core" (called the *powerhouse* by Pilates practitioners) includes the abdominals, pelvic floor, buttocks, hip, and lower back muscles. During a class, you strengthen these muscles, build muscular endurance, and learn how to initiate movement from this powerhouse. This helps support your knees, which can both prevent knee injuries and alleviate current knee pain.

"The knee is often a victim and not the cause of the knee problem. You have to look at the whole lower body, including the ankle, the hip, the low back. If your hip or ankle doesn't move well, this puts an extra load on the knee," says Stott Pilates instructor-trainer Kristi Quinn, of Bodycenter

Studios in Seattle, Washington. "If you are not using your low body correctly, Pilates can help retrain your body."

Chronic knee pain patients or people recovering from an acute injury or surgery can work with a Pilates instructor as part of their rehabilitation. Pilates is also an effective therapeutic practice for osteoarthritis sufferers. For these needs, find an instructor trained in rehabilitation and with experience in working with people with knee issues.

Working on Pilates equipment takes the pulling force of gravity off the knees, which can be vital if you are healing from surgery or have other more severe knee problems. For example, an instructor can lead an osteoarthritis patient through a series of gentle motions that eases pain and doesn't add wear and tear to the joint. "The equipment can support your [body]. You have resistance that you are pushing and pulling against to give you some feedback. It gives you information about your body," says Quinn.

Not all Pilates classes feature work on machines. Some classes use only mats—participants practice Pilates on exercise mats, using the effects of gravity. For someone with knee pain, this may be difficult. Try a machine class or one-on-one machine sessions first, and ask the instructor if or when you might be ready for a mat class.

Rumor has it that practicing Pilates also makes people taller. This doesn't mean you grow taller. This idea has its basis in better postural traits learned through practice. Pilates also builds leaner and longer muscles. If you choose to lift weights and become a bodybuilder, this adds bulk to your frame. Pilates has the opposite effect. "I think the changes [that make people seem taller] come from body awareness, core strength, and pelvic and spinal alignment that inevitably lead to better posture," says Thompson. "We do dozens of easy chores that can be done with a mind–body connection or not.

If I choose to engage my abdominal muscles and not lock my knees when I am picking up a stack of books, I will be making a healthy choice for my body that will benefit me and protect my back and my knees from unnecessary stress."

This mindfulness and better postural alignment carries over into everyday life. Maybe you walk with your shoulders rounded and your low back tucked in an irritating position. Through a Pilates practice, you'll begin to walk with your shoulders back and relaxed, and your low back in a more comfortable position, correcting poor postural traits and eliminating the corresponding knee pain. You'll learn to initiate muscles before you do some movements: before you get into a squatting position for gardening work, for example, you'll engage the muscles you need to do the movement correctly, without hurting your knees.

Finding a Pilates Instructor

As with yoga, there is not one unified certification process in the United States for Pilates instructors and trainers. When you check out a studio, it is important to ask if the instructors have undergone a training and certification process. There are numerous teacher-training programs, all with their own interpretations of Joseph Pilates's original regimen. If you are using Pilates as a rehab tool, find a practitioner trained in rehabilitation and with experience in working with people with knee pain issues. Ask the potential instructor the following questions about her certification process:

- How many hours of training were involved in actual practice? If she has trained for 900 hours, a majority of her training should be from doing Pilates as opposed to listening to someone talk.

- Did her training address knee issues, or does she have advanced training in working with knee issues?
- Did she learn anatomy and how to do postural assessments on her students?

One way to find a reputable studio is to call your local professional dance company and ask where the dancers practice Pilates. There are studio and instructor locators on the Internet as well; log onto the Balanced Body Pilates or Stott Pilates websites (see "Resources," at the back of this book).

Most Pilates studios have new students take one-on-one classes with an instructor. Each studio has its own rules concerning the number of individual classes students must take before they join a class setting. Executing a Pilates's movement correctly involves breathing correctly, tensing the right muscles, and moving in a controlled manner. You can practice Pilates without paying attention to these specifics, but your practice will lack the mind–body benefits, and some of the physical benefits. When you have ongoing knee issues, it's vital to move with a teacher's input guiding you. The teacher should be checking your postural alignment, asking you how you feel as you move, and paying close attention to how you move. If you are taking Pilates as a form of rehabilitation after a knee injury or surgery, expect the teacher to send you home with exercises to do every day. When your teacher feels you are ready for a group class, she will be able to direct you to the appropriate one.

If you are taking a regular Pilates class, set up a home practice by meeting privately with an instructor. If you buy home equipment, he can help you set it up and create an exercise regimen with you. As with an at-home yoga practice, creating three fifteen to twenty minute daily practices will help keep your routine interesting and allow you to put the practices together for a longer at-home session. See your instructor again when you are ready for a new routine.

THE FELDENKRAIS METHOD

Your knee issues may be resolved through learning new postural and movement habits. The Feldenkrais Method is a movement education program that aims to ease chronic pain and tension, and prevent acute pain flare-ups. Learning this system of gentle movements can improve your flexibility, balance, coordination, and posture.

Dr. Moshe Feldenkrais (1904–1984) developed the Feldenkrais Method after suffering from recurring knee injuries. Through his own self-awareness movement program, he was able to rehabilitate his knee. He was more interested in how well someone moved than in how perfectly he or she could sit or stand. Dr. Feldenkrais coined the term *acture* to reflect this idea. Optimal acture is the ability to move in any direction without preparation. When a Feldenkrais practitioner looks at someone sitting or standing, the practitioner evaluates how those patterns likely reflect the ways the person performs daily or recreational activities.

Picture a Barbie doll. She can't move well because her trunk is immobile. While other types of therapists might focus on helping Barbie achieve core strength, a Feldenkrais practitioner would help Barbie integrate her arm and leg movements with the movements of her midsection. Barbie's large muscles, joints, and small muscles should work cooperatively together. A Feldenkrais practitioner can help you identify your own habits of posture and movement, teaching you how to move in a more efficient and effective way.

If you see a Feldenkrais teacher for a one-on-one session—this is called a Functional Integration session—she will evaluate your postures and your movement patterns, assessing how these habits contribute to or even keep you in pain. She would choose hands-on techniques and exercises to help reduce symptoms. If you see a practitioner while you have an acute knee injury, she will place you in a comfortable posture that supports your knee and helps alleviate the pain. Working with your breath while you are in a posture will help your body become more relaxed; this also eases pain.

Even if your pain isn't 100 percent relieved through the Feldenkrais Method sessions, you will learn how to move smarter, be self-aware of the habits that cause pain, and gain self-care skills during sessions. You can also join group sessions, called "Awareness Through Movement" classes. During a class, if a movement doesn't feel good, make the movement smaller, or do it in your imagination. Even imagining the movement can help train your body to do the movement, since brain messages precede actions.

A reputable Feldenkrais Method practitioner should have completed a Guild Accredited Training Program—this takes roughly three to four years—through the Feldenkrais Guild of North America (turn to "Resources").

THE ALEXANDER TECHNIQUE
Like the Feldenkrais Method, the Alexander Technique (AT) is based on the idea that physical problems are linked to your posture and body movements. In the 1890s, Australian Shakespearean actor Frederick M. Alexander

created this method to cure his performance-linked laryngitis. Improving his head and neck posture put an end to his recurring ailment. The movement therapy Alexander developed focuses on how the head sits on the body; this is called *primary control*.

If you see an AT practitioner to help relieve your knee pain, she will use hands-on coaching and exercises to help you learn more optimal ways of sitting, standing, and moving. Although this is a popular movement therapy for actors and musicians, research also shows benefits for people with chronic pain.

You can study the Alexander Technique in a group class or in one-on-one sessions with a teacher. Your practitioner will examine your posture in various positions, watch how you move, and take note of your breathing patterns. As you learn how to move in ways that ease tensions, the practitioner may guide you with his hands. Learning AT will take varying amounts of time for each student, but ten sessions are often recommended. Find a practitioner who is registered with the American Society for the Alexander Technique; to qualify, practitioners must have trained for at least three years, undergoing a minimum of 1,600 training hours (see "Resources" for more information).

FINDING A SPORTS MEDICINE PHYSICIAN

If you are unable to remedy your knee pain through self-care or by learning a movement therapy, a trip to your primary care provider might be in order. (If you suspect you have one of the six most common knee injuries for adults—patellofemoral pain, MCL or ACL injuries, meniscal injury, osteoarthritis, patellar tendonitis/tendinosis, or iliotibial band syndrome—see your doctor to confirm your diagnosis.) Perhaps your doctor is well versed in musculoskeletal issues and she can treat your problem without a referral to another care provider. Often, though, your doctor will refer you to a physician who specializes in sports medicine.

Your doctor's advice on a suitable sports medicine physician is often the only advice you will need. However, you'll still want to make sure the sports medicine doctor is board-certified by the American Board of Medical Specialties (ABMS), which means he has gone through training and passed national board exams (see "Resources"). Make sure the sports medicine doctor is affiliated with a reputable hospital, as well.

If you are unable to get a referral from your doctor's office, or you want a second opinion, ask friends and family for the name of their favorite sports medicine doctor. You can also go online and look for doctors. Visit the American Medical Society for Sports Medicine. If you are specifically looking for a surgeon, log onto the American Orthopaedic Society for Sports Medicine. (See "Resources" at the back of this book for more information.)

When you visit a sports medicine physician, you should feel comfortable asking about his credentials. Does he specialize in knee problems and does he have experience with your injury? Make sure the specialist listens to you, as well. You'll want to tell the specialist how your injury occurred, what noises you heard or feelings you experienced when you injured your knee, and how you felt after the injury.

As discussed earlier, any doctor you see should be interested in you as a whole person. Looking at your entire life can guide your treatment. How has the knee injury affected your life, and what activities do you want to participate in after your knee heals? The doctor should want to treat any ailments with your input, talking about your goals and your responsibilities. For example, if you see a physical therapist, you will complete daily exercises. Perhaps you need to lose weight for surgery or to help with a chronic condition; this means you'll need to commit to a diet and exercise regimen.

THE ROLE OF PHYSICAL THERAPY

Often your primary care provider or sports medicine physician will prescribe appointments with a physical therapist. Physical rehabilitation is usually necessary after knee surgery. A doctor's referral often ensures that your insurance will pay for this therapy, but some states do allow patients to see a physical therapist without a doctor's prescription. Physical therapists have studied physical rehabilitation and work with patients who have illnesses or injuries that limit their ability to move their bodies and perform both daily and leisure activities.

Physical therapists (PTs) approach knee problems from a functional point of view. Your PT will develop a treatment plan that aims to improve your ability to move, reduce pain, restore function, and prevent disability, according to the American Physical Therapy Association. Your physical therapist will also help you build strength, endurance, power, and coordination of the muscles and other connective tissues in the knee joint and the rest of the body.

Picking a Physical Therapist

Often, your doctor will recommend a specific physical therapist. Several organizations can also point you in the right direction. Using the American Physical Therapy Association's consumer website (see "Resources"), you can locate physical therapists by geographical location or by their advanced specialty degree.

Some physical therapists are trained in the *McKenzie Method*, also known as *Mechanical Diagnosis and Therapy*. These physical therapists perform an initial patient assessment that looks at how pain and symptoms relate to your movements; the therapist then uses this information to create a treatment plan. Another goal of McKenzie Method–trained therapists is to teach you how to be in control of your own knee issues, so you can take care of yourself. You can locate a McKenzie Method–trained physical therapist at the McKenzie Institute's website (see "Resources").

It's helpful to work with an experienced physical therapist. This doesn't mean you need to seek out someone with twenty-five-plus years of knowledge. Instead, if your physical therapist is a recent graduate, ask if he is working in a clinic with a mentor program, where newer therapists seek guidance from more experienced therapists.

You'll be seeing your physical therapist a lot, sometimes twice a week or more. You will want to feel comfortable with this person. Larger physical therapy offices often have assistants; you'll spend time with the physical therapist and part of each session with the assistant. Make sure you are at ease with the assistants as well, and that you can see the physical therapist when you feel it is necessary.

The First Appointment

If you have never seen a physical therapist, you may wonder how this appointment will be different from a doctor's appointment. Every patient is unique, so the physical therapist won't be deciding on a treatment plan simply by reading your MRI or asking about your doctor's diagnosis. The physical therapist will ask you questions about how your pain behaves and how it changes with your positions, movements, emotions, and social situations. The appointment will be very physical. The physical therapist will watch you move, observing how you sit, walk, and stand, and even your preferred sleep positions. Most importantly, the physical therapist will actually touch your body, both while you are in motion and at rest, to see how your body's parts move together and to check for injury as well as strength.

The physical therapist will also ask you what activities your knee pain has forced you to curtail. The answers to this question will vary widely. Maybe you want to roughhouse with your children without wincing with pain, or you need to find a better way to work at your computer or a more comfortable sleeping position. Perhaps you want to run five times a week again, or rejoin your Wednesday night basketball league. Whatever these goals are, they will guide your physical therapy sessions. Your physical therapist will create an exercise program to strengthen your knee so that playing with your kids is fun again, you can set up your computer station without experiencing pain or injury, or you can adopt an exercise program that leads to running or playing three-on-three basketball.

Physical Therapy Modalities

Physical therapists may use one or more *passive therapies,* or *modalities,* to help treat your injured knee. Generally, the patient *receives* this treatment, meaning she is not actively involved in the treatment. Some physical therapists use these passive treatments sparingly, preferring patients to be as actively involved as possible in their recovery. Still, these modalities may help ease pain and promote healing. Often physical therapists use these modalities to treat the discomfort associated with acute pain or the acute flare-ups suffered by chronic knee pain patients.

- **Heat** or **cold packs** can help relieve your pain. A cold pack eases inflammation and decreases muscle spasms, while heat packs enhance blood flow. You can use heat or cold therapy at home. Rate your pain on a scale of zero to ten, with ten being the worst pain. If your knee pain is a three in the morning, but grows to a six in the evening, this is most likely a sign of inflammation. Treat your pain with an ice pack. If your pain stays a steady three throughout the day and night, use a heat pack. Some doctors don't recommend using heat for knee pain, unless it related to osteoarthritis. Over-the-counter Thermacare heat packs also can increase blood flow. These can alleviate hurt while sleeping, during long car rides or airplane trips, or during athletic activities.

- **Electrical stimulation** uses electrical current to cause a single muscle or a group of muscles to contract by putting electrodes on the skin. The muscles are either gently or forcefully contracted. This modality is often used for flare-ups of pain, sometimes in conjunction with an ice pack. Electrical stimulation can also help retrain muscles and nerves to work together to move.

- **Transcutaneous Electrical Nerve Stimulation,** or **TENS,** also uses a low level of electrical stimulation (which does not stimulate contraction of the muscles) to disrupt an unrelenting pain cycle by temporarily blocking a pain message. Often used for chronic pain, TENS is not a curative. Some therapists use TENS in tandem with exercise therapy, and recommend learning how to ease pain through a cognitive behavior modification therapy program.

- **Ultrasound** is a short, deep-heat therapy that uses high-frequency sound waves. This eases hurt, increases circulation, and relaxes tissues and muscles for a short duration, but at a deeper level than a heat pack.

- If you have a hard time doing land-based therapy, due to weight or movement issues, you may participate in **water therapy**. You'll complete exercises during active water therapy. When you are in a pool, gravity seems to no longer exert a force on your body. If you have severe knee pain, this can make it easier for you to complete movements. As you begin to heal, you may transition from water to a land-based regimen.

- **Braces** are temporary fixes for people who experience excessive pain while moving in certain ways. A brace restricts movement while you learn muscle control and postures to ease this pain. This modality is often used after surgery. Some people always wear some form of a knee brace while participating in certain athletic endeavors.

- **Manual medicine** and **massage therapy** relieve pain and stimulate a healing response. Your physical therapist may use these modalities when you plateau, meaning you are not getting any better or worse, to help jump-start the therapeutic process. The physical therapist or massage therapist uses their hands to localize the force on deep tissues and joints of the body. (For more information on massage therapy, turn to Chapter 7.)

Exercises and Physical Therapy

The bulk of each physical therapy appointment is about movement. The physical therapist will create a stretching and exercise regimen to address your knee's specific problems. Although each regimen is unique, often a patient will work on:

- Postural and gait issues. Strengthening muscles to support your knee joint, including the quadriceps, hamstrings, and abductor muscles, the iliotibial band, the buttocks muscles, and the low back and abdominal muscles. Other muscles you might work on: the gastrocnemius, which is a calf muscle, and the popliteus and plantaris knee muscles.

- General aerobic conditioning to build your endurance, bring oxygen to the tissues, and elevate your mood.

- Strength and resistance training to build the overall strength of your knee and body.

- Relearning daily activities and sports techniques, so you can perform them in ways that don't harm your knees.

Your physical therapist is trying to improve the perceivable deficits caused by your knee issues. This will mean performing exercises during appointments and doing exercises on a daily basis. Your physical therapist will break the exercises into steps or stages, teaching you how to perform each movement correctly, down to breathing techniques. The exercises shouldn't provoke symptoms, but you can expect soreness, similar to the pain you would feel from completing any exercise regimen. You'll learn how to move with the least amount of pain possible during your daily life and while participating in your favorite leisure activities.

6 PRACTICES FOR THE MIND

STUDIES ABOUND ON THE BENEFITS OF MEDITATION.
According to various reviews, meditation can help lessen anxiety, mild and moderate depression, excessive anger and hostility, insomnia, and high blood pressure; prevent heart attacks; and ease the symptoms of PMS, menopause, and arthritis.

Few studies have examined knee pain and meditation, but numerous studies have looked at the effects of meditation on chronic pain patients. Mindfulness meditation had numerous benefits for the chronic back pain patients who took part in an eight-week study reported in *Pain* in 2008. (Mindfulness is one type of meditation practice.) These patients experienced less pain, improved physical function and pain acceptance, and better sleep. Such relief would be most welcome to people suffering from knee pain.

Another study, reported in *NeuroReport* in 2006, showed that people skilled at meditation had a 40 to 50 percent lower brain response to pain than people who did not practice meditation. The people in this study practiced transcendental meditation, a mantra-based meditation practice. After the initial research was gathered, the nonmeditating participants learned transcendental meditation. Five months later, these twelve participants were retested. Now that they had practiced meditation, their brain responses to pain had also dropped by 40 to 50 percent.

With both an acute knee injury and chronic illness such as osteoarthritis, the experience is not just about the physical pain, but also about your response to pain. The story you tell yourself about the hurt can help lower your pain level, or this tale can take the discomfort to the level of infinity. Even without changing the level of physical pain—you can make a tremendous positive impact on your symptoms by simply changing your reaction to the pain and creating a more positive story about your injury or illness and your life. This can lower the amount of pain you feel, lower your medication usage, and improve your quality of life.

WHAT IS MEDITATION?

Practicing meditation evokes the relaxation response, which lowers metabolism, blood pressure, heart rate, and breathing rates. Essentially, while you meditate, you calm your mind and slow down your body, creating balance and a sense of wholeness.

During meditation, you relax your logical mind, and then you access the part of the brain that is driving your subconscious. The subconscious is what you are acting from when you automatically respond to a painful fall from your bike or when you yell at your arguing children. You can think of meditation as giving your conscious self a nap, so you can talk positively to the subconscious mind. The way you talk to your subconscious depends on what type of meditation you practice. For example, with guided imagery, you envision what you want to happen. Some types of meditation use an

MASTERING MINDFULNESS AND EASING PAIN

Keep in mind that learning any form of meditation takes time, even if it is a movement therapy such as yoga or tai chi. You may give up too soon, not realizing this skill takes time and persistence.

Meditation is weight training for the mind. Think about preparing for a physical endeavor. You plan on climbing Mount Rainier or hiking twenty miles of the Appalachian Trail. You begin hiking smaller amounts every weekend, taking daily walks, and lifting weights at the gym. You cross-train by practicing other sports; you eat healthy foods; and you make sure to get plenty of sleep.

There is no way you could summit Mount Rainier or complete your Appalachian hike without plenty of preparation. The mind works the same way the body works. The first time you practice meditation, you won't automatically master it. Learning how to meditate takes practice, persistence, and discipline.

If you practice a form of meditation on a daily basis, you start to bring that frame of mind to your entire life. A strong meditation practice can help you recognize the moment where you get to decide how to react. When you feel your knee ache as soon as you try to get out of bed in the morning, you can decide how to react. You can take five deep breaths, and respond with calmness. Instead of thinking how your whole day will surely be horrible now, you can think of strategies that will help you feel better or how you can arrange your day to work around the pain. You may lessen your pain through your deep breathing and intention to stay calm. At the very least, you might react more calmly to the situation, decreasing stress so you can avoid tensing up your muscles, which is a contributor to your knee pain.

affirmation or mantra to program your mind with positive thought. Meditation that involves movement might have you focus on a positive intention while you move.

By focusing on your breath and body, you place yourself in the present moment. This breaks the train of everyday thought, putting aside the past and the future. This momentary lapse from your life—whether it's ten minutes once a day, or twenty minutes twice a day—has the power to help you rest deeply and feel better. Meditating is a skill you can learn that helps you focus on positive thought and on what you want to happen in life.

STRESS AND THE BODY

Think about how you respond to a stressful situation. Thanks to your knee pain, you have a hard time getting ready for work. The extra minutes it takes to get out of bed, put on clothes, make your breakfast, and walk your dog around the block have already put you behind schedule. Your knee and leg muscles, ligaments, tendons, and connective tissue—which were already hurting—tense up even more.

Then you encounter horrendous traffic on your way to work. You react immediately, without thinking: your body tenses even more, and your knee pain intensifies, turning from a dull throb to hot pain. You curse and your shoulders are so tight they almost touch your ears.

When faced with stress, your body responds via a built-in fight-or-flight mechanism: your metabolism, blood pressure, heart rate, rate of breathing, and blood flow to the muscles increase.

"We secrete stress hormones, but we neither run nor fight," says Dr. Herbert Benson, director emeritus of the Benson-Henry Institute for

MUSIC THERAPY

Listening to music can evoke the relaxation response. After composer, musician, and meditation practitioner David Ison broke his back, he created an acoustic therapy program to help himself walk again. Now called the TheraSound Method, a study published by the National Institutes of Health in 1999 documents this music program's ability to elicit the relaxation response. The participants—272 patients suffering from chronic pain problems—lowered their pain an average of 54 percent through this method.

After Ison injured his back, he noticed that meditation brought a reduction in pain and improved his concentration, which helped foster his healing. The music he created for TheraSound replicated the breathing pattern of meditation. People who listen to these compositions breathe in time to the music, which evokes the relaxation response in their minds and bodies. While you can simply listen to TheraSound music as a form of therapy, you can also listen to these compositions while practicing other forms of meditation, using the sounds to help develop your practice. You can purchase acoustic therapy music by contacting TheraSound (see "Resources").

Mind Body Medicine at Massachusetts General Hospital, and author of *The Relaxation Response.* "Stress is related to over 60 percent of visits to the doctor. No drugs or surgeries effectively treat this. Fortunately, just as we possess the fight-or-flight response, we as humans also have within us what's called the relaxation response. It is the biochemical, physiological, and genetic opposite of the fight-or-flight response."

Most of us don't realize we actually have a split second to think about how to respond to our stress. Usually we automatically behave based on how we have reacted in the past, according to the patterns we learned long ago. In that moment, we are actually at a place of choice. We can decide how to react. Meditation is a way of training the mind to recognize that moment, so we can respond in a way that is less stressful and more empowering.

MEDITATION BY ANY OTHER NAME

Meditation can be any type of activity that elicits the relaxation response in a person. Dr. Benson, one of the first doctors who connected meditation and Western medicine in the United States, coined the term *relaxation response* in the 1970s. He notes that all humans have the ability to evoke this calming body response, and you can choose the technique that works best for you.

Dr. Benson defined one relaxation response method, but this is just one of many types of techniques. Usually a method involves repetition, such as a word, a sound, a prayer, a phrase, or movement. One technique isn't better than another technique. Other forms of meditation include transcendental meditation, mindfulness meditation, tai chi, repetitive prayer, and walking meditation.

Practicing any movement therapy that has you focus on your breathing while moving your body with intention can be a meditative experience, including yoga, Pilates, or physical therapy exercises performed with meditative focus. If you have trouble sitting still, try yoga, tai chi, or

PREPARING MENTALLY FOR SURGERY

Studies show that relaxation techniques, positive thinking, and guided imagery and visualization practices not only help you prepare for surgery and post-operative recovery, but also increase your chances of a successful outcome and a faster recovery. One program that has proven particularly effective was developed by psychotherapist Peggy Huddleston and is described in her book *Prepare for Surgery, Heal Faster: A Guide of Mind–Body Techniques*. Huddleston, a psychotherapist, recommends the following five steps as a means of preparing for surgery:

- Relax to feel peaceful.
- Visualize your healing.
- Organize a support group.
- Use healing statements.
- Establish a supportive doctor-patient relationship.

Her book and the accompanying CD (or tape or MP3 file) guide you through each step.

Forty-four people who both took part in Huddleston's workshop and used her techniques before and after knee replacement surgery had less anxiety on the day of their operation and left the hospital 1.3 days sooner than the patients who did not use these techniques or attend the workshop, according to an unpublished study on Huddleston's website (see Resources). Huddleston's procedures can also be used to make your post-operative recovery process easier, faster, and more successful.

In Chapter 9, the sections "Mind–Body Surgery Preparation" and "Post-Surgical Life" describe in detail Huddleston's steps and materials; please turn to those pages for complete information.

walking meditation. If you like quiet, learn transcendental or mindfulness meditation.

With meditation, daily practice is the key. Practicing once a day is better than not practicing at all, meditating ten minutes twice a day is even better, and twenty minutes twice a day is the ideal.

The Relaxation Response Technique

The relaxation response method is easy to learn. Before you try it, pick a word or phrase to use during practice. This word, thought of as an affirmation, should be positive. If your word or phrase has a sacred component, it's called a mantra. Remember this means the word is sacred to you as an individual. Using a mantra can elevate a meditation practice, because the word is even more positive than an affirmation. Essentially, this word is programming your subconscious mind with positive thoughts. Examples of affirmations and mantras include "one" and "peace."

Now that you have your word, find a quiet place and sit down in a comfortable position. Close your eyes and focus on relaxing the muscles in your body. If this is hard for you, try starting at your toes and relaxing your body, part by part. Then focus on your breathing. Breathe in slowly. As you breathe out, say your affirmation or mantra. Let's use the word "peace" as an example. Breathe in. Exhale while saying, "Peace." Continue doing this for ten to twenty minutes.

If you become distracted and other thoughts enter your mind, simply say, "Oh, well." Then return to your repetition, breathing in, and then exhaling while saying, "Peace." When you are done, open your eyes and sit for another minute or two. Practice the relaxation response twice a day. That's all there is to this simple method.

If Dr. Benson were leading the relaxation response for you, he might count your breaths at the beginning and end of your practice. Usually your breath rate would slow by a handful of breaths or more, proving the relaxing effects of this technique.

Transcendental Meditation

Dr. Benson studied transcendental meditation for his original research on the relaxation response. He realized that transcendental meditation, like many other meditative practices, elicited the relaxation response. There are numerous studies on the benefits of this form of meditation for anxiety, depression, and pain. To learn more about this technique, visit the Transcendental Meditation Program's website (see "Resources" at the back of this book). Learning transcendental meditation usually involves a seven-step course taught by a certified teacher. Go to the Transcendental Meditation Program's website to find a class near you.

A Mindfulness Practice

Mindfulness meditation stems from the Buddhist meditation tradition. Dr. Jon Kabat-Zinn began teaching Mindfulness-Based Stress Reduction (MBSR) when he founded the University of Massachusetts's Stress Reduction Clinic in 1979. The goal of mindfulness is to cultivate awareness of the present moment.

Eight-week MBSR classes are now taught at the Center for Mindfulness in Medicine, Health Care, and Society, an outgrowth of the original clinic, and at more than four hundred locales around the world (see "Resources" at the back of this book). You can learn mindfulness meditation on your own. Unlike the relaxation response, mindfulness doesn't use an affirmation or mantra. Participants focus only on the breath. To practice mindfulness, find a quiet spot. Then:

- Sit in a straight-backed chair with your feet flat on the floor, or sit on the floor.
- Relax. You can do this by focusing on relaxing the muscles in your body, from your feet to the top of your head.
- Focus on your breathing: on the flow of air around your nostrils; on the feeling of the breath as it goes in and out; and on your belly as it rises and falls according to your breathing.
- If your mind becomes distracted, just come back to focusing on your breaths.
- Keep focusing on your breaths for twenty minutes.

By practicing mindfulness—or any type of meditation—for twenty minutes, twice a day, you are learning how to be aware of the present moment, and learning how to focus your mind. With these skills, you can begin to be aware of that moment in time where you get to choose how to respond to an event in your life, such as that traffic jam on your way to work. If you usually react to a bout of pain by getting angry and thinking your whole life is terrible due to your knee, you can meditate with the intention to change this reaction. Next time you feel that familiar pain, you can focus on breathing deeply and staying calm. You can say to yourself, "Yes, my knee hurts, and this is horrible right now. Still, in general, my life is good. How can I lessen my pain and still enjoy the rest of the day?" Meditation is training the mind to be in the present moment, both during practice and in your daily life.

Guided Imagery or Visualization

If you have never meditated, guided imagery or visualization is an easy-to-learn meditation style. You'll use your imagination to visualize a positive outcome.

To practice:

- Sit comfortably.
- Relax your body. You can do this by focusing on relaxing the muscles in your body, from your feet to the top of your head.
- Relax your conscious mind by focusing on your breathing for a while.
- Imagine a positive outcome for your ailment or problem. For knee pain, you could imagine light going into your knee and healing it. For changing how you react to traffic jams, focus your intention on changing your reaction to the inconvenience of modern life. Think of options for responding to the traffic jam while you meditate: breathing deeply, listening to soothing music, and realizing that your commute time is out of your control. You can focus your intention on ways to react to bouts of knee pain as well, which may very well include the same tools as responding to the traffic jam.
- Practice this twice a day for twenty minutes.

You can buy guided imagery and visualization tapes, CDs, and DVDs. These can be helpful tools if you are new to meditation or if you are looking for structured guidance. The Benson-Henry Institute offers guided relaxation CDs online, along with relaxation response method CDs (turn to "Resources"). Some yoga classes have a guided imagery component. You can also look for guided imagery and visualization classes in your community.

Walking As Meditation

If you like to move, walking meditation might be a good fit for your life-style. If you cannot remember the last time you sat still, try this method. Mindfulness guru Dr. Kabat-Zinn has his students walk in circles in a room or back and forth in a lane while learning walking meditation. To practice walking meditation, follow tips culled from Dr. Kabat-Zinn's book *Full Catastrophe Living: Using the Wisdom of Your Body and Mind to Face Stress, Pain, and Illness*:

- While walking, focus on sensations in one part of your body. Beginners can focus on just their feet or just their legs. Be aware of each foot or leg as it moves.
- Add in an awareness of your breathing as you walk.
- If you lose focus and your mind wanders, just bring your attention back to each foot or leg as it moves, and again focus on your breathing.
- Focus your gaze in front of you instead of looking at your feet or at the sights around you.
- You can walk at any pace, slow or quick.
- Practicing walking meditation alone is a way to be less self-conscious about learning it, and can help with focus.
- While you are learning walking meditation, practice it for short periods, perhaps five or ten minutes.

As you become an adept meditative walker, you won't need to walk in circles or back and forth from wall to wall. You can practice walking meditation for longer periods of time, maybe even for miles on an outside trail. After you are adept at concentrating on just one body part, try focusing on your whole body and its sensations.

7 BODYWORKS

HANDS-ON THERAPIES CAN BE INCREDIBLY HEALING. Called *bodyworks*, these modalities are numerous and varied. A bodywork therapy may be an integral part of your care plan. Adding one or more of these complementary practices to your medical care may enhance healing, ease pain, and promote a sense of wholeness.

Sometimes it is hard to imagine how bodyworks fit into medical care. Perhaps you haven't heard of some of the therapies discussed in this chapter. Not all of these practices are understandable in Western medical terms. Some techniques focus on *meridians*—invisible energy channels that you will not find in a Western-style anatomical drawing. This doesn't mean such techniques won't be beneficial for your specific knee issues.

Think of medical care options we've talked about throughout this book as a wheel—the spokes represent the plethora of health-care options available to you, including bodyworks. Stepping onto the hub, you are in charge of your medical care, gathering information and working with knowledgeable practitioners who listen and see you as a whole person.

What bodyworks therapies might help alleviate or even prevent future episodes of knee pain?

Sometimes a practice won't be the right fit for you or for your knee problem. If you try a bodyworks therapy and don't find any relief or see any progress after a handful of sessions, it might be time to move on. This can be discouraging. Still, it's worthwhile to try new paths to healing, whether that means trying a different bodywork technique or talking to your knee specialist about other options.

It's also helpful to think about the term *healing*, which isn't defined by a cure. "*Healing* implies the possibility for us to relate differently to illness... as we learn to see with eyes of wholeness," writes Jon Kabat-Zinn, PhD, in *Full Catastrophe Living*. There isn't always a complete cure for knee pain, but you can begin to see yourself as a whole person with knee pain. Healing may mean learning self-care methods to alleviate your pain, seeing a bodyworks practitioner and your doctor as needed, and living your daily life as fully as possible. Your path to healing is a unique journey. Read on to learn more about bodyworks therapies.

MASSAGE

Massage is an ancient, manual, hands-on therapy (although a practitioner may apply pressure to your body with other body parts, from his elbows and forearms to his knees and feet). Hippocrates, often called the father of medicine, wrote this in 460 BC: "The physician must be experienced in many things, but assuredly in rubbing."

Today, more than eighty types of therapies fall within the category of massage. These manual therapies treat the body's muscles, ligaments, joints, skin, and connective tissues. Various types of massage attempt to affect whole systems of the body, including the lymph nodes, and the gastrointestinal, musculoskeletal, circulatory, and nervous systems. At the very least, you may have some level of muscle tightness or guarding due to your knee pain. Massage helps relax the body. Massage can be a holistic therapy, treating the mind, body, and spirit. The human connection inherent in massage fosters a sense of well-being and wholeness.

Picking a Massage Style or Therapist

How do you find the type of massage that is right for you and your specific condition? Picking a type of massage is similar to picking a yoga style. The yoga style you choose is dependent on the expertise of the teacher leading the class. "Any system of massage that lasts long enough to be well-known is likely to have value, but that value is only as good as it is artfully applied by the practitioner," says Wolfgang Brolley, a massage therapist and physical therapist who practices in Seattle, Washington.

Any practitioner whom you see for your knee problem is likely to have massage-therapist recommendations. Ask friends and family if they have received an excellent massage from a local therapist. It's not as easy to find a massage practitioner by looking online, but it can be a good starting place. The National Certification Board for Therapeutic Massage & Bodywork (NCBTMB) certifies massage and bodywork practitioners (see "Resources" at the back of this book). To receive this accreditation, a therapist must show mastery of a core skill set, pass an exam, uphold the NCBTMB's standards of practice and code of ethics, and take part in continuing education programs. Currently, forty-three states regulate massage therapists, and several states have pending legislation. Ask your potential therapist if he or she has accreditation through your state or a local governing board.

Obviously, a lengthy discussion of every style of massage would merit a book of its own but we'll discuss several types of massage. Most of the bodyworks practices in this chapter also fall within the massage category. For a more thorough list of styles with accompanying descriptions, look online at Massage Today, a web-based massage therapy publication (turn to "Resources").

When you imagine a massage, you are probably picturing *Swedish massage.* Known as classic massage in Sweden and parts of Europe, this style originated during the eighteenth century in Sweden. Considered the most common massage type, Swedish massage incorporates five basic strokes— long gliding strokes, kneading, striking or tapping, vibration or shaking, and rubbing—to work the muscles and connective tissue. This relaxing style of massage lessens pain, improves circulation and range of motion, and helps to detoxify the body's tissues. When your body's muscles are tense, chemical waste products stagnate, causing irritation and pain; Swedish massage helps eliminate this waste. Swedish massage is the underlying technique for several other massage styles. *Deep tissue massage* focuses on loosening up the deepest muscle layers. *Sports massage* uses techniques from both Swedish and deep tissue massage to prevent injury and to aid in healing after injury occurs. Athletes also use sports massage to keep their bodies in optimal condition for competition.

Therapeutic Massage from A to Z

We won't cover every letter in the alphabet, but the following types of therapeutic massage may relieve your knee pain.

- *Acupressure* therapists focus pressure on the anatomical points used in acupuncture. Instead of needles, therapists use their hands to restore flow to invisible energy channels called meridians. For more information on this massage style, see this chapter's "Acupuncture" section.

- *CranioSacral therapy* (CST) works with the membranes that surround the brain and spinal cord, called *dura mater*. According to CST therapists, these membranes have a slow but palpable motion or pulse; CST therapists can feel this pulse throughout the body. Disturbances or blocks in this pulse negatively affect your nervous system. A CST practitioner restores this pulse.

- Physical therapists often use *myofascial release techniques* on patients. Fascia are the connective tissues that envelop the entire body. If you removed all the other matter in the body, this spider web of tissues would still create the structure of your body. Myofascial release finds the areas of your body where the fascia is stuck, scarred, or immobile. The therapist applies slow and steady pressure to these tissues, promoting healing.

- *Reflexology* operates from the principle that reflex points on the hands and feet correspond to points on the rest of the body. Reflexologists use massage and pressure on the hands and feet to encourage healing at various places in the body. Some practitioners also work on a patient's ears.

- *Shiatsu* technically means *finger pressure*. During this Japanese massage style, the therapist uses massage techniques on the invisible energy channels, or meridians, of your body. Instead of using needles, as in acupuncture, shiatsu practitioners use their thumbs, fingers, palms, and/or feet to massage you.

- Dating back more than 2000 years, *Thai massage* actually has its beginning in India. Depending on training, therapists use a combination of gentle massage, acupressure, stretching, and placing patients in positions similar to yoga poses.

- Trigger points are painful areas, bands, or knots in muscles. In the 1940s, Dr. Janet Travell mapped the body's trigger points. During *myofascial trigger-point therapy,* a practitioner locates the trigger points that need release, uses pressure to relieve the point, and usually massages the area after this release.
- Stemming from Chinese medicine principles that date back centuries, *tuina* (*twee nah*) aims to restore flow in blocked or stagnant energy channels. During a treatment, the practitioner applies massage techniques on anatomical points, meridians, muscles, and nerves.
- A French osteopath pioneered *visceral manipulation. Viscera* means organs, and this type of massage focuses on imbalances between your organs and corresponding body structures. For example, pain that shoots down the front of the leg can be a referred pain from one of your organs.

THE BOWEN TECHNIQUE

Created by Australian Thomas Bowen in the 1950s, this soft-tissue technique has several monikers, including Bowenwork, Bowen therapy, and Bowen Technique. A Bowen therapist uses a stretch-and-roll-through technique. By stretching tissues, she challenges the tissues for a brief moment, then moves over that point in a perpendicular fashion, and creates a muscular release, as well as sending a neurologic message to the brain that helps the body recharge. Bowen believed the body has a natural ability to heal itself, and that his technique helped the body reset itself.

During a Bowen session, the therapist will actually leave the room from time to time, giving each body section a few minutes to begin responding to the moves. The Bowen Technique works in a sequential way to help the whole system. Therapists believe Bowenwork returns the body to a state of homeostasis.

If you see a Bowen therapist for a knee problem, she will do a physical assessment, checking your posture and looking for muscular and connective tissue restrictions anywhere in your body. The therapist will work to release the tension in the primary site of pain, as well as addressing issues in the entire body. Although the number of sessions varies, you can expect marked improvement after three to four sessions; many patients say they feel an overall sense of well-being. If you have chronic knee pain or compensatory postural positions have developed over the years, a longer period of therapy may be necessary.

ROLFING

Rolfing has a beginning similar to countless other therapies and exercise regimens. Ida Rolf created this soft-tissue manipulation and movement education program because she was seeking solutions for her and her sons' medical ailments. (Coincidentally, Ida Rolf earned her PhD in biochemistry in 1920, the same year all women in the United States were granted the right to vote.)

Dr. Rolf coined the term *Structural Integration* for her deep-tissue massage therapy program. Today, people commonly call her technique Rolfing, although the formal name is "The Rolfing Technique of Structural Integration." Dr. Rolf believed that the connective tissue holds the body together and gives us our shape. Picture your connective tissue as a spider web linking all the body parts; this web would still hold your body's structure even if everything else in your body was removed. Dr. Rolf believed that as we age, our connective tissue becomes misaligned, as well as less elastic and tough, placing demands on the rest of the body and causing poor postural traits. Rolfers use a variety of pressures to manipulate the fascia. This realigns the body structure within this connective tissue, helping to correct postural traits and balance the body within gravity.

If you see a Rolfer for your knee pain, he might suggest undergoing what is called the Ten Series, a standardized recipe of Rolfing. A Ten Series practitioner will aim to systematically balance and optimize both the structure and movement of your entire body by the end of ten sessions. During your first visit, the practitioner will look at your body as you stand and as you move. Your Rolfer will apply pressure to your body with his fingers, knuckles, and elbows at the level where the connective tissue begins to release. This can be an intense experience, and Rolfing might feel painful at times. Rolfers believe the patterns that can cause pain in the body are not only physical, but emotional as well. Rolfing frees up both physical and emotional restrictions. You may cry, or laugh, or have other emotional reactions to this physical therapy. Sometimes practitioners recommend a form of psychological therapy to help with these issues. The time between sessions—sometimes weeks or even months—gives your body and mind time to process the therapy and integrate the physical, emotional, and psychological changes into your life.

Practitioners don't always prescribe the Ten Series; you may have a handful of visits or a dozen appointments. You may see a reduction or a complete alleviation of pain through this therapy. You can also expect to learn better postural traits and become more aware of your body. Rolfers are licensed through the Rolf Institute of Structural Integration (see "Resources" at the back of this book).

HELLERWORK STRUCTURAL INTEGRATION

Joseph Heller, the founder of Hellerwork, was actually the first president of Dr. Ida Rolf's Rolf Institute. Branching off from Dr. Rolf's work, Heller further addressed the spiritual and emotional aspects of the mind and body. Along with structural integration bodywork, Hellerwork includes movement-posture education and body-centered dialogue.

As with Rolfing and other forms of Structural Integration, a Hellerwork practitioner uses deep-tissue massage to restructure your body's fascia. This releases tension, allowing changes in posture and movement patterns. Movement education is intrinsic in each session. You will learn new ways to sit, stand, and move through the practitioner's touch and guidance. The practitioner and client acknowledge and discuss ("dialogue about") the psychological issues that come up during a session. The dialogue component stems from the belief that our emotions manifest themselves in our bodies and their movements.

Hellerwork sessions explore the psychology of "selves," examining the idea that every person has multiple selves or parts. Because of a person's personal history, certain aspects of a person's personality tend to come to the forefront, becoming a central aspect of how she lives her life. This in turn influences the person's posture. Let's say the "pusher aspect" of someone's personality is strong; that is, she *pushes* to get everything done. This aspect of her personality isn't interested in relaxing in Hawaii. Hellerwork strives to help a person notice such dominant parts or selves, as well as opening the patient up to other aspects of her personality. By bringing conscious awareness to your entire personality, Hellerwork aims to give you more choices, leading to a fuller life. Joseph Heller calls this the "coming home to your body" principle.

Your first visit to a Hellerwork practitioner will involve the same physical assessment as used by other bodyworks practices: the practitioner will observe your body's structure, posture, and movement patterns. Hellerwork has an eleven-session series designed to realign the body systematically while releasing chronic tension and stress. For example, the first session focuses on the theme of inspiration. This session centers on the rib cage, breath, and what inspires you and fulfills your spirit. While these are the jumping-off points for this appointment, each patient and session is unique. Your practitioner may prescribe a different number of sessions based on your specific needs.

A certified Hellerwork practitioner has graduated from a Hellerwork International School, is licensed and insured, partakes in continuing education workshops, and follows a professional code of ethics and standards (turn to "Resources" for more information).

OTHER STRUCTURAL INTEGRATION THERAPIES

Besides Hellerwork, numerous other bodyworks therapies stem from Dr. Rolf's original work. These practices are based on the idea that gravity, everyday life, injuries, movement patterns, and attitude can affect your body structure, leading to pain. As in Rolfing and Hellerwork, practitioners of these other therapies use massage techniques to restructure the body's fascia and overall physical structure. Depending on the type of Structural Integration practice, a session may also include movement education. Emotions and behavior patterns may also be addressed. Each type of Structural Integration practice looks to balance the whole person. You can find Structural Integration practitioners at the International Association of Structural Integration website (see "Resources"). This site includes links to

HYPNOTHERAPY

If you can recall the sensation of falling asleep, you are familiar with the state of hypnosis. Just as you start to drift off to sleep with your eyes closed, yet while you are still aware of sounds, feelings, and sensations, you are passing through a state of hypnosis. Similarly, when you wake in the morning, you are aware of the sounds of birds, the feeling of somatic sensations in your body, and although your eyes are still closed, you are aware of the room being lit by soft, morning light. Once again, you are coming through a state of hypnosis. We experience trance or hypnosis many times during the day. Meditation and hypnosis share some common traits, while still being quite different. Meditation has a more

open-ended focus, while a trance state has a more focused awareness. While you are in trance, your conscious mind steps aside, allowing the unconscious mind to step into the spotlight. An important note: all hypnosis is self-hypnosis. Even though the hypnotist is "inducing" a trance, the practitioner has no power or control over the subject.

Hypnosis has a long history in the field of pain management. The National Institute of Health has officially endorsed it as an effective treatment for pain alleviation. Hypnosis can also lower your heart rate and blood pressure, and lead to relaxation. If you need surgical intervention for your knee problem, it's also an effective way to lessen pre-surgical anxiety and lower post-surgical pain and complications.

Seek a practitioner with experience in using hypnosis for pain management. During your appointment, the hypnotist will take a complete medical history. Then the practitioner will explain hypnosis with a pre-induction talk. The trance state develops through the building of rapport and various techniques. Helping you achieve a deep state of trance is accomplished in several ways, including progressive relaxation, eye fixation, eye opening and closing while counting backwards, arm catalepsy, and confusion inductions.

Once you have achieved trance, the hypnotist uses techniques that involve various suggestions, images, and unconscious learnings to teach you how to be pain free, or, at the very least, how to control uncomfortable sensations in your body.

Although there is no national standard licensing system for hypnotists, the largest organization for health and mental health-care professionals using clinical hypnosis in the United States is the American Society of Clinical Hypnosis (ASCH). You can find a hypnotherapist on the ASCH website (turn to "Resources").

several bodyworks organizations, such as the Soma Institute of Neuromuscular Integration, the Institute of Structural Medicine, and Kinesis Myofascial Integration.

CHIROPRACTIC CARE

Chiropractic therapy works with the biomechanics of the backbone to restore function to the body. The spine's top twenty-four vertebra connect above and below, and each one of these connections can move in six different ways. A lack of movement or flexibility in a joint can cause pressure on the joint and the surrounding tissues, perhaps irritating the nerve roots and putting nearby muscles into spasm. A chiropractor maneuvers and massages the spine joints—a process called *spinal manipulation*—aiming to restore full mobility to the specific joints and body.

"Chiropractic care is an art form on top of a diagnostic skill. You have to find the joint that is restricted or locked, and then use your hands-on skill to help the patient gain full function," says Lew Estabrook, a Seattle-area chiropractor. "Similar to a surgeon, the chiropractor has to have good diagnostic skills with good techniques to get effective results. If one chiropractor does not solve a health issue, do not give up. Try a second chiropractic opinion."

Finding a skilled chiropractor is important. Ask friends, family, and your other practitioners for referrals. A licensed chiropractor has completed a minimum of two years of pre-med courses and then graduated from a four-year academic chiropractic program and passed state or national exams, earning a doctor of chiropractics, or DC, title.

During your first visit, the chiropractor will take a thorough history of your systemic problems, and you will undergo a movement-oriented examination. Some practitioners always take X-rays or other diagnostic images, while others order imaging only for some patients. During an adjustment or treatment, your practitioner will use a variety of hands-on techniques to put pressure on the joint or joints. Often literature on chiropractic care talks about a cracking or popping noise that signals repositioning. This is just one technique, and your practitioner may not use this style of care during a visit. Even if your chiropractor uses this high-velocity technique, your body may not have an audible response. The goal of treatment is to restore more normal function to the joint, taking pressure off the surrounding muscles, ligaments, and nerve tissue. This gives your body an opportunity to go through its normal healing process.

Every chiropractic patient has a unique schedule of appointments, but you should see some results after a handful of visits. As your body begins responding to treatment, often your chiropractor will have you do exercises and stretching to help restore strength and stamina to your knee, back, and body. Similarly, your chiropractor may recommend other types of care to help with your knee-pain issue. Some chiropractors may recommend adjustments on an ongoing basis, although no studies have shown a benefit for seeing a chiropractor for long-term treatment. Look for a practitioner who has a clear timeline for treatment, with an end in sight.

OSTEOPATHY

Osteopathic doctors also practice spinal manipulation. American physician Andrew Taylor started osteopathy after concluding that the musculoskeletal system is fundamental to the health of a person's body. While osteopathic doctors have learned Western medical practices, they also have studied osteopathic manipulation and holistic health practices. While seeing an osteopath is similar to visiting an MD, treatments can also include:

- Osteopathic manipulation
- Physical therapy
- Movement and exercise education
- Nutrition
- Reducing stress through relaxation techniques

As opposed to chiropractic care, which tends to focus on manipulating the spinal column, osteopathic manipulation addresses the entire musculoskeletal system. Like other bodywork practices, osteopathic medicine aims to put the entire person into balance: mind, body, and spirit. By seeing a doctor of osteopathy, or DO, you can seek both conventional treatments as well as a range of complementary therapies (listed above). To learn more about osteopathic medicine or to find a DO in your area, log on to the American Osteopathic Association (find this information in "Resources").

ACUPUNCTURE

It's safe to say acupuncture is one of the oldest medical practices still used in the world today. The earliest known records state that acupuncture grew out of Wu Shamanism in the Shang Dynasty with the first needles fashioned out of bone. As acupuncture has evolved over a 5,000-year period, it has been influenced by various cultures, as well as Taoist, Buddhist, and Confucian philosophies. While acupuncture has progressed and changed, the art remains rooted in traditional models and theories that have been tried and tested in clinical applications.

Acupuncture aims to restore the flow of *qi* in a patient's body. *Qi* (pronounced *chee*) is a living dynamic that, for lack of a better word, is often translated as "energy." In theory, the qi courses through the human body via pathways called meridians or channels. When there is an obstruction (stagnation), excess, or deficiency of qi—due to trauma or changes in your body—this balance is upset. This produces physical discomfort that can manifest itself as pain in your body, whether that pain is local or throughout an entire system in your body.

If you see an acupuncturist for your knee pain, you will be treated for both the presenting symptom (pain), and the root cause of the imbalance. The acupuncturist may employ several traditional methods of examination to determine the root cause, including taking a complete medical history, a pulse diagnosis, abdominal diagnosis (called a *hara diagnosis*), facial diagnosis, tongue diagnosis, and also looking for signs of blood stagnation and swelling if there is knee pain due to trauma. The acupuncturist should be conversant with Western medical protocol as well. After the exam, the practitioner will weave together a diagnosis based on what is presenting at the time.

As treatment begins, the practitioner selects pre-sterilized filiform needles that are made from stainless steel. These needles are inserted locally at the site of the injury, as well as distally along the channel pathways. Many people wonder how much acupuncture hurts. Often people say that it is painless or that inserting needles hurts

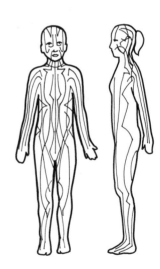

7.1. Meridians or Channels

as much as yanking on a single hair, although not quite as much because the needles are so thin. The acupuncturist may also choose a form of heat therapy called *moxibustion*, in which the herb mugwort is either burned on the head of the needle or applied directly to the skin. This produces an increase in the flow of blood and qi systemically and locally in the body. Where there is stagnation of blood, the application of cups (a process called *cupping*) can be used to break up adhesions and old stagnation. As acupuncture is a "hands-on" form of therapy, bodywork and massage are also employed. Acupuncture naturally increases the circulation of blood, lymph, and qi in the body. This relieves your body of discomfort and allows your body to restore its own healing properties.

A course of acupuncture treatment usually takes between five to ten sessions, depending on the severity of the injury, how long the problem has been in the body, your age, and your constitution. Usually you will not need to get fully undressed, but simply roll up your sleeves and your pant legs. Sometimes you'll need to get undressed down to your underwear. Each session takes about an hour.

Some doctors are trained in acupuncture. There are different state requirements for doctors obtaining an acupuncture degree; you'll want to verify that your doctor holds a certified state license. Practitioners who aren't MDs obtain a masters degree in acupuncture and undergo a comprehensive accreditation procedure through the National Certification Commission for Acupuncture and Oriental Medicine (NCCAOM). Locate an acupuncturist online at the NCCAOM website, or by logging onto Acufinder.com, an online resource for acupuncture, Chinese herbs, and Asian medicine (see "Resources").

8 FOODS, HERBS, AND SUPPLEMENTS

"YOU ARE WHAT YOU EAT" is a common expression, but what does it really mean? When you have knee pain, is there a direct stomach–knee connection? Maybe that candy bar you ate for a snack wasn't the best choice, but can it really intensify your knee pain?

Inflammation often causes pain and swelling. If you cut your index finger while chopping onions, your finger usually doesn't hurt very much at first. A day or so later, though, your cut and the somewhat swollen area around it feels much worse. That's because your body's defense system, otherwise known as your immune system, started an inflammatory process to heal the cut. The chemicals sent to heal your injury are actually irritating the nerves around the cut.

Sometimes this inflammatory response is too strong, causing even more pain. Let's say your brain is sending chemicals to repair a sprained MCL in your knee. This inflammatory-response team sends cells to the area to help it repair, but the chemicals the cells release can irritate the nerves, which causes more pain. If the response is too vigorous and goes on too long, it can result in scarring, which makes your knee joint less flexible and more prone to injury the next time you play basketball.

You can modulate your body's inflammatory process through diet, supplements, and herbs. Through simple changes, you can decrease your likelihood of generating an overly high inflammatory response. This may not only ease the pain caused by your knee injury, but may also positively affect other health issues related to inflammation.

HOW DIET HELPS

You need your body's inflammatory-response system to live. Without it, even that simple finger cut wouldn't heal. Sometimes, however, the inflammatory-response system over-reacts. Imagine dropping a wine bottle on the floor and watching it shatter. Instead of picking up the pieces yourself, you call a fire squad and a police team, along with a hundred friends to clean up the mess. All of these people would end up creating a bigger mess in your kitchen than any shattered wine bottle. In like manner, your inflammatory-response team can worsen a problem.

Through changing your diet, you can help regulate your inflammatory process. Several elements in the diet determine the level of your inflammatory response, including types of fat in your body as well as the amount of antioxidants and phytochemicals available for your body to use.

Fatty acids are the building blocks of fats. Our bodies cannot make essential fatty acids. We obtain fatty acids from the food we eat. Fatty acids change the type of chemicals your body's immune system secretes during an inflammation reaction. By changing the types of fats you consume, you can change the level of inflammation you experience. Two types of fats that are essential for our bodies are omega 6 and omega 3 fats. Most Americans consume too much omega 6 fat in comparison to omega 3 fat. This imbalance promotes inflammation in the body. You can decrease inflammation by increasing your intake of omega 3 fat to balance the ratio of omega 6 to omega 3.

Antioxidants are compounds found in foods, especially in fruits and vegetables, which quench the inflammatory response and protect tissues from damage by blocking free radicals. Free radicals are unstable compounds generated in the inflammatory process that can damage DNA and cells.

Phytochemicals are compounds found naturally in plants that have numerous health benefits, including anti-inflammatory ability. Examples of phytochemicals include flavinoids, which are often found in berries. Flavinoids may actually deactivate enzymes that promote inflammation.

Below are diet suggestions that can help to regulate your immune system, so the next time your knee pain flares up, there is less pain and swelling during the healing process and a smaller chance of scar tissue forming. Following these guidelines will balance the amount of omega 6 and omega 3 in your body, as well as the amount of oxidants and antioxidants.

EAT THESE FOODS
Want to help decrease inflammation in your body (and in your poor aching knee)? Here's a primer on types of food to include in your diet. Eating these healthy foods is an easy way to possibly lower your pain level and decrease your immune system response the next time you suffer a bout of knee pain.

ADDITIONAL SUPPLEMENTS FOR OSTEOARTHRITIS

If your knee pain stems from osteoarthritis in the knee joints, taking the following supplements may help relieve pain, improve movement, and help repair cartilage in the joints. (Again, ask your doctor before taking any supplements.)

Research shows that taking *glucosamine sulfate* can be more beneficial than taking nonsteroidal anti-inflammatory drugs (NSAIDs) such as ibuprofen. Most studies look at osteoarthritis and the knee, showing many benefits for patients. Unlike NSAIDs, glucosamine sulfate helps repair cartilage, and study patients experience fewer side effects than participants taking NSAIDs. A study in Portugal showed benefits for 95 percent of the participants with knee osteoarthritis; benefits included less pain while resting, standing, and exercising. Take 1500 milligrams once a day. Be sure you purchase the sulfate form; this type of glucosamine has more data supporting its usage than the other form, called glucosamine hydrochloride.

Patients may see more benefits by taking glucosamine sulfate with *chondroitin sulfate.* This supplement may alleviate pain from osteoarthritis and help repair damaged cartilage. Take a daily dose of 1200 milligrams.

Osteoarthritis sufferers may also see symptom improvement while taking *niacinamide* supplements. However, this supplement may cause liver damage and problems with blood sugar. If you wish to take this supplement, do so under strict supervision by your physician.

Cold-Water Fish

The acronym *SMASH* stands for salmon, mackerel, anchovies, sardines, and herring. Try to include these types of fish in your meal plan. Partaking in the fish associated with SMASH is a good starting point for including fish in your diet, but eating any type of cold-water fish may have anti-inflammatory benefits.

Fruits and Vegetables

Increase your daily intake of fruits and vegetables. Although all fruits and vegetables have anti-inflammatory properties, try to include the ones with the darkest pigments. Deep-colored fruits and veggies have more plant pigments and vitamins per bite, which contain antioxidants. Berries—blueberries, raspberries, blackberries, strawberries—have the most benefits for your body. Likewise, the greenest vegetables are your best bet, such as broccoli, spinach, and winter greens. These substances can actually de-activate enzymes that promote inflammation.

Whole Grains and High-Fiber Foods

Add whole grains and high fiber foods to your menu. Whole grains and high-fiber foods balance your insulin response. There is a relationship between your insulin response and your inflammation. When you eat sugar, a hormone called insulin increases. If you eat refined sugar, you get a larger insulin response in comparison to eating a small amount of sugar while also consuming a whole grain or high-fiber food. Having chronically high insulin levels is associated with increased inflammation.

When you are buying grains, look for the color brown. Choices include brown rice, whole grain breads, whole grain pastas, spelt, buckwheat, and barley. Learn how to cook these grains from whole foods or vegetarian cookbooks, such as *Vegetarian Cooking for Everyone* (see "Bibliography" at the end of this book.) High-fiber foods include fruits, vegetables, and whole grains. Other examples include beans or legumes. Add any legume to your weekly menu: lentils, split peas, and garbanzo, red, pinto, and black beans.

Water

You have heard it before, but we will say it again. Drink more water. Aim to drink eight glasses of H_2O every day.

AVOID THESE FOODS

Parallel to the list of foods to include in your diet are foods to decrease or avoid. The following foods can increase inflammation, leading to more pain. Minimize these food types in your menu plan.

Red Meat and High-Fat Dairy Products

Red meat and high-fat dairy products such as cheese and whole milk have a type of fat called *saturated fat,* which promotes inflammation. It is best to reduce these foods in your diet. If you still want to eat red meat, limit your intake and try to buy grass-fed meat, which is better for your body.

Sugar

Avoid refined sugar, including white sugar, brown sugar, and high-fructose corn syrup. All sugars impair the functioning of your immune system. Even sugar in its natural form—molasses, honey, and maple syrup—should not be a regular part of your diet.

White Foods

Take white foods off your recipe ingredient list. Try to remove white flour, white bread, and white rice from your pantry.

Flavored Drinks

Don't be swayed by flavored bottled waters. Take a pass on any flavored drinks, including soda pop, vitamin-style waters, lemonade, and juice. You want to avoid these sugar-laden drinks.

Processed Foods

Avoid processed foods. Buy whole foods, meaning products that have not undergone extensive manufacturing processes. Fruits, vegetables, and whole grains have had little done to them before they reach your local grocery store. Foods with ingredients labels that include hydrogenated oils or artificial sweeteners are far from their natural states.

HERBAL SUPPLEMENTS

Some herbal supplements can modulate or balance the inflammatory process happening in your body. Taking the supplements and herbs described below may decrease the pain associated with knee problems. Ask your doctor before taking any supplements. Some medications may interfere with these products, and certain medical conditions may limit the types of supplements and herbs you can include in your diet. Just like taking over-the-counter and prescription medications, you may suffer side effects while taking herbal supplements. If you are going to have surgery, you may need to stop taking some of these suggested supplements two weeks before your operation; again, ask your doctor.

Fish Oil

Besides eating cold-water fish, take a daily dose of fish oil. Look for this in the refrigerated section of a supplements store, your local health-food market, or even in your neighborhood grocery store. In a comprehensive summary study that reviewed the data of several other studies, patients who took fish oil for at least three months had less self-reported pain, less morning stiffness in their joints, fewer number of painful joints, and were able to reduce the use of non-steroidal anti-inflammatory drugs (NSAIDs). Take two capsules of fish oil daily, each with 1000 milligrams of omega 3 fat. Look for brands that have been independently tested for mercury and other contaminants. Molecularly distilled forms of fish oil are better for you because they are more likely to have had contaminants removed during this process. Use the website ConsumerLab.com to look for brands that have been independently reviewed (see "Resources" at the back of this book). Stop taking fish oil two weeks before any surgery. If you are currently taking a blood-thinning medication, talk to your doctor before starting a fish-oil supplement.

Curcumin

Curcumin comes from turmeric plants. Used for generations in India, it gives curry its yellow color. Of greater importance, curcumin is an antioxidant with anti-inflammatory properties. Take 400 milligrams of curcumin three times a day. This substance absorbs better if you take it alongside a fatty food or if the product is in gel-cap form. (Supplements in gel-cap form are in an oil base.) Curcumin may work better if you are also taking bromelain, described below.

Bromelain

Bromelain is a mixture of enzymes from pineapple. Studies show this agent lessens inflammation, bruising, and swelling after sports injuries or other traumas. In a study published by *Practitioner* in 1960, seventy-four boxers took bromelain. Within four days, bruising cleared up in fifty-eight boxers, while the rest of the boxers needed eight to ten days for all signs of bruising to disappear. Seventy-two boxers didn't take bromelain. Within this group, just ten participants had no bruising after four days, and the rest of the group needed seven to fourteen days for the bruising to dissipate. For the best results, take bromelain while also taking curcumin. Buy bromelain that is standardized to 2000 mcu's per 1000 milligrams. Take 500 milligrams three times a day, between meals. *Caution*: avoid if allergic to pineapple or if you are on a blood thinner or have liver problems.

Ginger

Perhaps ginger already flavors some of your dinner entrees. This botanical has anti-inflammatory and antioxidant properties. Take two to four grams of dry, powdered ginger or about a half inch of sliced, fresh ginger daily; you can simply incorporate it into your vegetable dishes. Taking ginger may thin your blood, so talk to your doctor if you are already taking a blood-thinning medication.

Boswellia

The herb boswellia comes from the gum resin of the *Boswellia serrata* tree, which is native to India. Most commonly used as a treatment for osteoarthritis, this herb has anti-inflammatory properties. Look for boswellic acid extracts and take 300 milligrams three times a day. *Caution*: avoid if you suffer from heartburn.

9   WESTERN MEDICAL INTERVENTIONS

YOU DIDN'T THINK YOU WOULD END UP HERE. You're accustomed to trekking up trails full of switchbacks, paddling across lakes, or running up and down a soccer field twice a week. Now, just the idea of getting out of bed is causing you anxiety. This morning you were worried that your right knee would give out when you tried to stand up.

Before today, your knees had rarely given you trouble. If one of your knees hurt after a long training run or a rugged hike, you took ibuprofen, iced and elevated your knee that evening, and spent a few days reducing your activity load. But the pop you heard and felt during yesterday's soccer match clearly wasn't a minor injury. It's time to call your doctor. You think you tore your ACL. You wonder if surgery is in your near future.

The first ACL repair surgery took place in 1895. Replacement ACL surgery followed, with the initial attempt—using braided silk—occurring in 1903. Today, routine ligament reconstruction surgeries for torn ACLs are more than 82 percent successful. Still, not every ACL tear needs surgery. You'll need to review your options with care.

If self-care methods aren't alleviating your pain from another common knee problem—patellofemoral pain, osteoarthritis, tendonitis, IT band syndrome, a meniscus tear, or an MCL tear—it's time to explore other options. Medications and medical procedures are often Western medical treatments. It's important to approach medical care with caution. Taking charge of your own health care includes making an informed decision about your available options. Read on to learn about medications, injections, and surgical interventions, as well as how to prepare for an operation.

MEDICATIONS 101

Unless your injury is severe—with pain greater than a six on a zero-to-ten pain scale—and/or you are experiencing any red flag symptoms (see Chapter 2), doctors recommend self-treatment using the R.I.C.E. method: rest, ice, compression, and elevation. You can use these four components to ease swelling and pain and promote healing. (Read about the R.I.C.E. method on page 37, in the box "R.I.C.E.: Knee Injury Self-Care.") Supplement the R.I.C.E. procedures with over-the-counter (OTC) medications to bring more relief from pain and discomfort.

OTC Medications

Although OTC medications are readily available, that doesn't mean they can't have potentially dangerous side effects. Always read and follow the label on your OTC medications. If you take OTC medication for an injury for more than a week, it's a good idea to get your doctor's opinion. She can alert you to side effects, and let you know the best possible regimen for your injury. Sometimes patients need to take tests to check for potential side effects of OTC medications.

Following are brief descriptions of both OTC and prescribed pain-management medications.

- OTC pain relief medications are also called *analgesics*. The term *oral non-steroidal anti-inflammatory drugs,* or NSAIDs, is a catchall phrase for a variety of medicines that ease stiffness and pain while reducing inflammation. If patients use NSAIDs for an extended period, possible side effects may include stomach ulcers, or liver and kidney problems. OTC NSAIDs include aspirin, naproxen, and ibuprofen; common brand names for some of these drugs are Motrin, Aleve, and Advil.

- Acetaminophen, with the common brand name Tylenol, alleviates pain as well. For some people, acetaminophen doesn't offer as much pain relief as OTC NSAIDs, but it has the benefit of fewer side effects. (Keep in mind, however, that high doses of acetaminophen can damage your liver.)

Topical Medications

You can apply topical analgesic creams, sprays, or rubs to your skin. Some creams contain salicylates, the main ingredient in aspirin. You also can choose a cream with capsaicin in it; these creams block pain messages to the brain by stopping a neurochemical called substance P from transmitting pain and inflammation signals. Apply most topical medications several times a day. Don't use these creams under a compression bandage or wrap, or while using a heating pad.

Prescription-Level Pain Relief

If OTC medicines don't alleviate pain or you need to take pain relievers for an extended period of time, your doctor can prescribe prescription-strength NSAIDs. Patients typically experience fewer gastrointestinal side effects while

AN ACL STORY

Lisa Sicchio McKenny was playing soccer, but her injury could have just as easily occurred while she was running in the park with her kids. She was sprinting in a straight line, and then she started to cut to the left. McKenny's foot stayed planted and the upper part of her leg twisted. "I knew instantly I had torn something. I heard a pop, felt serious pain, and saw it almost dislocate as it happened," says McKenny. She had a torn ACL and a big bone bruise.

Her knee was completely unstable after the tear: It felt wiggly and as though it was going to give out. McKenny could walk in a straight line with no problems, but if she tried to turn or run, she felt her knee would not hold itself together. She underwent an ACL repair surgery that used a hamstring tendon graft. After a successful surgery, she had a leg-bending machine delivered to her house.

She spent two full days having the "Constant Perpetual Motion" machine bend her leg back and forth. She was in serious pain and had swelling for roughly a week. She wore a brace for six weeks and did physical therapy for three months. After six months, stay-at-home mom McKenny was jogging and feeling pretty good. "The knee was still really stiff and I felt like I would hurt myself if I played soccer. I started back at soccer fifteen months after surgery," she says.

Today her knee feels good, but she is timid about cutting and running at full-sprint speed. McKenny has no knee pain, although her joint now cracks—similar to when you crack your knuckles. She still completes her physical therapy exercises every day. Her injury and surgery haven't stopped her from participating in anything, but she doesn't play as rough anymore.

taking NSAIDs called cyclooxygenase-2 inhibitors (COX-2). Take prescription-level medications at the lowest possible dosage for the shortest period, under a doctor's care. Some studies show that some COX-2 drugs might increase an individual's risk for cardiovascular events. Tramadol or Ultram are also prescribed for pain relief; these drugs lack the side effects associated with both NSAIDs and acetaminophen, but they can still be sedating, cause seizures, and have narcotic-like effects.

Your care provider may recommend narcotic, or opioid, medications for acute pain. This type of medication deadens a person's pain perception. Side effects may include sedation, nausea, constipation, itching, sweating, and muscle twitching. Long-term use may have a risk for addiction or abuse, so any long-term usage needs to be well thought-out and executed with close monitoring by your doctor. Often patients take opioids for just a one- or two-week period.

NEEDLES AND THE KNEE

Only a few conditions call for sticking a needle in your knee, according to Dr. David Belfie, an orthopedic surgeon who practices in Seattle. If a knee is swollen, a needle aspiration can be performed to extract some of the fluid for analysis. (Findings may include blood, joint fluid with crystals in it, or infections.) Patient comfort is another reason for a doctor to draw fluid from your knee. If your joint is uncomfortably swollen due to osteoarthritis or a knee injury, your doctor may recommend a needle aspiration.

Reasons to inject medications into the knee are few. Corticosteroid injections calm down an inflamed knee joint. These injections, which are also known as steroid or cortisone injections, are most often used for painful flare-ups of osteoarthritis. Steroids can also be injected for bursitis and iliotibial band syndrome. Usually cortisone injections are not used for patellar tendonitis; even though cortisone has anti-inflammatory effects, there is a risk of rupturing the tendon. Usually the knee is aspirated first, removing excess fluid from the joint. For arthritis, pain relief from steroid injections should last at least two to three months. Most knee specialists recommend having this procedure done just two to four times a year. If you are prescribed steroid injections more often than this, you have an increased risk for weakening tendons and softening cartilage, which is why most doctors avoid it.

If you are in pain due to a lack of articular cartilage—the protective connective tissue that covers the ends of the bones surrounding the knee joint—your doctor may recommend a dose of hyaluronic acid substitute, called viscosupplementation. Osteoarthritis is also the main reason for this type of injection. Hyaluronic acid is one of the building blocks of articular cartilage; this fluid helps lubricate and cushion the knee joint. The fluid used in viscosupplementation is usually derived from rooster combs. The cost of this treatment is significant, even with medical insurance.

As with any medical procedure, steroid injections and viscosupplementation have possible side effects and complications. Sometimes there is increased swelling or pain for the first day or two after an injection. An infection is another possible side effect; signs of infection include fever or excessive pain, swelling, or redness.

WEIGHING THE SURGICAL OPTIONS

Unless you need emergency surgery for a knee trauma, you have time to weigh your options. Take a deep breath if your doctor recommends visiting the operating room. Surgery isn't always the best option for each patient or

A TALE OF THREE KNEE INJURIES

When it comes to her knees, insurance consultant Karen Schuler is both ill fated and lucky. In less than a decade, she suffered a trio of knee injuries. She tore her meniscus around age twenty. Her knee was already sore from coming down on it wrong while playing basketball. Then she slipped on a wet staircase and twisted it. It hurt right away, but she recalls the pain was worse the next day. She had a sharp pain on just one side of her knee and the joint was stiff.

When Schuler was twenty-four, she had tendonitis in both of her knees. They felt stiff and tender and she had a hard time walking.

The tendonitis came on gradually. Her doctor said this injury was caused in part by wearing flat shoes such as Keds and ballet flats.

Finally, Schuler tore her ACL at age twenty-six. She twisted her knee while skiing, and knew immediately that she had hurt it. The pain was sharp and in a specific location.

Where does her good fortune come into this tale? Schuler didn't need surgical interventions for any of these conditions. The orthopedic doctor she saw for her meniscus tear talked about surgery as an option, but Schuler wanted to exhaust all other remedies first. Physical therapy was a good solution for all three injuries: the tendonitis, and the meniscus and ACL tears. Her physical therapy regimens consisted of riding a stationary bike and working on a stair climber, as well as completing exercises and stretches to increase her range of motion, build up the muscles around the knee, and keep those same muscles and her knee joints limber.

Since Schuler has suffered cartilage damage over the years, she works to maintain good muscle tone to keep her kneecaps in place and working well. More than ten years later, her knees rarely bother her. "They get stiff every once in a while, but that's probably due to my age. I limit how often I wear flat, unsupportive shoes like ballet flats, and I do weight-bearing exercise at least three times per week," she says. "When my knees start to bother me, I almost immediately head to the gym for stretching and a light workout. If I experience pain, I'll ice my knees before taking medication."

every single diagnosis. You'll want to investigate alternatives, trying some of the therapies mentioned in previous chapters before agreeing to a procedure. If surgery makes the most sense for your specific condition, you'll want to gather information and prepare yourself for the operation.

Although we hear about people having knee surgery all the time, we're usually hearing about just a few types of operations. Your cousin probably tore his ACL, and your next-door neighbor underwent meniscus repair. Still, before you decide on surgery for one of these conditions, be aware: even these common procedures are not always necessary.

What about all those sports stars undergoing knee operations? Beyond the torn ACL, competitive athletes have knee problems that the general population rarely encounters, so many of the surgeries are not common.

In Chapter 2, we discussed the seven most common knee problems affecting the average adult. Four of these conditions rarely require surgery:

- Patellofemoral pain, which is also called patellofemoral syndrome, anterior knee pain, or patellar chrondromalacia
- MCL injuries
- Tendonitis and tendinosis
- Iliotibial band syndrome

Below we'll discuss surgical options for the remaining three conditions: ACL injuries, meniscus injuries, and osteoarthritis. First, let's think about the attributes you'll be looking for in a surgeon.

Selecting a Surgeon

Many highly qualified surgeons perform knee operations, but not every one of them is the right surgeon for you and your condition. Even though your health insurance may limit your choices, make every effort to find a surgeon with whom you feel comfortable and who you feel is the most qualified to treat your particular knee problem. Ask your primary care doctor which surgeons he would recommend. Try to find family or friends (or friends of friends) who have had knee surgery and ask them for recommendations.

It is a good idea to interview at least two surgeons before making a decision, remembering that you are in charge of your medical care. Review each surgeon's qualifications during your appointment. Ask the surgeon how many times he has performed this specific surgery—this should be a routine procedure for him. Most importantly, do you feel comfortable with this surgeon? He may not have time to answer fifty questions, but he should answer a reasonable number of questions and you should feel that he listens to you. The surgeon should see you as an individual, with goals and a set of circumstances that are unique to you. Is surgery—or even a minimally invasive procedure such as an injection—the best possible fit for your life?

Don't Forget to Ask

Before you decide on a surgical intervention, make sure you have all the information you need to make an informed decision. When you are interviewing surgeons, ask the following questions:

- Do my diagnostic tests match the procedure the surgeon recommends? (This is another way of asking if the surgeon knows the specific cause of your pain.)
- What percentage of people have successful outcomes based on my specific diagnosis?
- Is this still an experimental surgery?
- What are the risks, benefits, and possible complications of this surgery?

- What are the pre-surgery preparations and how can I be in the best possible shape for this surgery?
- What will happen before the surgery?
- What happens during the surgery?
- What can I expect post-surgery and during recovery, both immediately at the hospital, and in the weeks and months following surgery?
- Will the doctor be available for consultation and follow-up after the surgery?
- Is the surgeon part of a care team that includes physical therapists and other types of practitioners that I will see after surgery? (In other words, will you and the surgeon create a comprehensive care plan?)
- What will physical rehabilitation involve?
- What nonsurgical treatments or therapies can I try before agreeing to surgery?

Tell the surgeon you are getting a second opinion. (The surgeon you are talking to should welcome another opinion.)

Perhaps most importantly, the doctor should be able to communicate clearly the risks and benefits of your procedure. He shouldn't see you as just another routine procedure. Instead, the surgeon should ask you about your specific set of circumstances. In addition, you should feel comfortable talking with the doctor; establishing a working relationship will help ensure the best possible outcome for your surgery.

ACL RECONSTRUCTIVE SURGERY

If you hurt your ACL, you are in good company: approximately 200,000 Americans injure this ligament every year. About half of these injured patients undergo ACL reconstruction surgeries. How will you know if you should opt for this surgery? If you've only partially torn your ACL and can continue with all of your daily activities after it heals, you may not need an operation. If you have completely torn your ACL, it is helpful to know how some sports medicine doctors decide on surgery for their patients.

Sports physicians often cite two main reasons for getting an ACL surgical repair. One is knee instability: your knee gives out when you stand on it or when you do simple maneuvers such as pushing your shopping cart around the corner of a grocery store aisle. Avid athletes who want to continue doing their high-risk sports activities also have their ACLs repaired. For example, soccer may be a big part of your life—even though you aren't a professional athlete, you play in two leagues a week. You may well opt to have surgery if you injure your ACL.

Even if you fall into one of these two categories (knee instability or avid athlete), you should consider factors such as the following before deciding on surgery. First, you will need support for the first few weeks after surgery; if you are unwilling or unable to take the necessary time off for the first few post-surgical weeks or if you don't have the support necessary for recovery, you should say no to surgery. Also, you need to be committed to completing as much as a year of physical therapy. Finally, you should make sure you don't have any medical health issues that would affect your ability to go through surgery.

You may be able to avoid surgery for an ACL tear if you are willing to give up your high-risk sporting activities and if you wear a knee brace for certain activities. If you don't have an ACL reconstruction surgery, you may still be able to resume exercising, though probably not at the same level. Remember, whether you undergo surgery or not, you will still need to participate

KNEE SURGERY FOR OSTEOARTHRITIS AND THE PLACEBO EFFECT

A study published in 2002 changed the way surgeons thought about surgical meniscal repairs for people suffering from knee osteoarthritis. Published by the *New England Journal of Medicine,* the study showed that sham surgery was just as effective as surgery that "cleans up" a patient's meniscus.

At the Houston Veteran's Administration Medical Center, arthritis patients were divided into three categories. The first group underwent arthroscopic debridement, which means the meniscus was smoothed and cleaned up, with tears trimmed, loose cartilage bodies removed from the knee,

and the joint irrigated and washed. The second group simply had an irrigation and wash, and their meniscuses were not touched. The third group had knee incisions made, but no surgical instruments entered the joint; these patients all had sham surgery. All of the participants were studied for two years after the operations. None of the patients knew which surgery they had received. All of the patients had some success, with less hurt and better knee movement. More people in the arthroscopic debridement group claimed the least amount of success. Surprisingly, the people who claimed the most success were often those who had undergone the sham surgery. (This is called the "placebo effect": people feel better simply because they believe they have received treatment.)

Overall, there was no marked statistical difference between any of the groups. Not only does this show the power of the mind over the body, but also that arthroscopic debridement surgery for osteoarthritis is often not an ideal choice. A 2005 study showed that 75 percent of thirty-two patients who had symptomatic osteoarthritis had meniscal abnormalities on their MRIs. Now patients who have symptomatic osteoarthritis and meniscal tears may choose to have meniscus surgery less often. If they do have this surgery, the pain from osteoarthritis will still be present after surgery. (The benefits of this knee surgery were also examined by a Canadian study published in 2008; see the "Osteoarthritis" section later in this chapter.)

in intensive physical therapy to strengthen your knee and prevent further injury.

There are a handful of types of reconstruction ACL surgery. Choose the type of surgery your surgeon recommends. He'll know what kind is best for your particular case and he'll be most comfortable performing certain types of operations as well.

After you tear your ACL, it's unlikely that you'll have surgery immediately. It's common to wait six weeks, so swelling can dissipate and the joint can calm down.

During an ACL reconstruction surgery, the torn ligament is replaced with a "new" ACL. This replacement ACL is created from an autograft or an allograft. An autograft is composed of the patient's own tissue taken from another part of his or her body; tissue choices can include the patellar tendon, or hamstring tendon. An allograft comes from a cadaver's tissues.

After an ACL repair operation, physical rehabilitation is essential. You'll meet with a physical therapist on a regular basis until you have regained full range of motion in your knee joint, and good balance and control in the entire leg. This can take as few as three months or as long as an entire year.

MENISCAL SURGERY

Surgeries to repair the meniscus are one of the most common operations performed in the United States. Surgeons liken the meniscal repair operation to a person trimming his fingernail with a nail clipper. Instead of using a nail clipper, the doctor uses a scope and longer instruments, but she is essentially trimming out the torn part while leaving as much meniscus intact as possible. If the tear is near the outer edge of the meniscus, the surgeon will instead stitch the torn parts back together.

Although this surgery has a high success rate for a good candidate, not everyone with a meniscus injury is an ideal candidate for this procedure. If you are under the age of thirty-five and don't suffer from osteoarthritis, meniscal repair can be highly successful, especially if the tear is in the outer portion of the meniscus where the blood supply is good. Your doctor may recommend surgery if you:

- Have trouble bending your knee (called a "locked" knee)
- Can't straighten the knee fully
- Hear a popping or clicking sound and experience knee pain

Most people over the age of thirty-five have some degree of mild cartilage wear or osteoarthritis in their knees. You may not even experience pain from this condition. However, if your MRI shows a torn meniscus and you have significant osteoarthritis, be wary about meniscus surgery. Unless there are mechanical problems—such as the ones listed above—surgery usually isn't warranted for this population group, and surgery may not even address present mechanical problems. Dr. Christopher Wahl, a team physician and orthopedic surgeon at the University of Washington in Seattle, believes a patient with a torn meniscus has at best a 50/50 chance of feeling better after meniscus surgery if he or she also suffers from osteoarthritis. This is because it's not possible to tell if the pain is coming from the meniscus tear or from the arthritis. If the pain is coming from both issues, you may get relief from the meniscus tear but you will still have pain from the osteoarthritis.

After meniscal surgery, recovery make take anywhere from three to six months. Physical therapy is an important part of the recovery process to restore function in the knee.

SURGERY FOR OSTEOARTHRITIS

Surgical procedures for osteoarthritis sufferers are a last resort. A procedure to smooth the meniscus and clean out the knee joint was common until a study published in 2002 showed that sham surgery was just as effective as real surgery (see the box "Knee Surgery for Arthritis and the Placebo Effect," in this chapter). This knee surgery, commonly called *arthroscopic debridement*, was also examined in a Canadian study published in 2008. Half of the Canadian study's patients had surgery, followed by physical therapy and medications. The other half of the participants received only physical therapy and medications. Three months after the first group had surgery, both patient groups experienced some success. However, the surgical group had no statistical advantage over the nonsurgery participants. The lead researcher felt the improvements experienced by both groups could be in part because of the physical therapy, follow-up care from nurses, and an in-home exercise regimen.

In other words, if you are suffering from osteoarthritis, approach arthroscopic debridement surgery with caution. If a doctor recommends this procedure because a person has a meniscus tear on top of the osteoarthritis diagnosis, the surgery might help alleviate the pain from the tear, but the arthritis pain will remain.

If you suffer from osteoarthritis pain, self-care is a big part of a treatment plan. Trying therapies mentioned in previous chapters can alleviate pain and help you avoid the doctor's office. Dr. Lawrence Holland, an orthopedic surgeon practicing in Seattle, recommends avoiding medical interventions for as long as possible. When that isn't possible, using anti-inflammatory medication is usually the first step of medical care. Cortisone or viscosupplementation injections are the next step.

If your aching knee becomes the focus of your life—and you are fit enough for surgery—a doctor may recommend a partial or total knee replacement. Still, these types of surgeries should be considered only if all other options have been exhausted. For the average adult, these types of surgical interventions are rare.

PREPARING FOR SURGERY AND RECOVERY

Patients who actively participate in their health care have better surgical outcomes than patients who are more passive. You can engage in the surgical process by gathering information about your surgery, asking all of your questions, and feeling comfortable with your surgical decision and your surgeon. Here are other factors to keep in mind when preparing for surgery:

- Try to be in the best physical shape possible for you. Smoking can cause complications, so quitting smoking four to six weeks before surgery is a good idea.
- Go over the medications and supplements you are currently taking with your surgical team. You may need to stop taking some of them before surgery.
- If you have other medical conditions, such as diabetes or hypertension, meet with the specialists you see for those conditions. You'll want to make sure all of your medical issues are under control.
- Plan for your recovery, with friends and family set up to help with your care after surgery.
- Know what to expect after surgery, from understanding how you might feel to how long your recovery might take.

- Make sure your post-surgery plan gives you enough time to recover, without returning to work or activities too soon.
- Be committed to post-operative rehabilitation.
- Be psychologically ready. You can take part in pre-surgery psychological screening and preparation if you or your doctor thinks this is necessary.

Mind–Body Surgery Preparation

Peggy Huddleston's book *Prepare for Surgery, Heal Faster: A Guide of Mind–Body Techniques* recommends five steps to help people prepare for both surgery and post-operative recovery. Huddleston, a psychotherapist, originally created these tools to help several of her patients have less fear while preparing for their own operations. It's best to start working on these steps two weeks before your surgery, but even if you complete the steps only one day before surgery, Huddleston believes you will still see benefits. Huddleston's five steps are:

- Relax to feel peaceful. The relaxation CD (or tape or MP3 file) that accompanies her book guides you through an exercise that will put you in a deep state of relaxation. Listen to this twenty-minute CD twice a day.
- Visualize your healing. Turn your worries into positive healing energy for your knee. The relaxation CD will guide you through this process, so you can picture yourself with a healthy knee participating in activities that you love. Again, this twenty-minute relaxation CD will guide you through this process twice a day.
- Organize a support group. Ask your friends and family to think of you with love for thirty minutes before your surgery. Patients who do this report feeling a sense of peace and love wrapping around them like a blanket.
- Use healing statements. Ask a nurse or your anesthesiologist to say three

healing statements. As you go under anesthesia, this person says, "Following this operation, you will feel comfortable and heal very well." Toward the end of surgery, this person says, "Your operation has gone very, very well." At the end of surgery, this person says, "Following the operation, you will be hungry for [your favorite white liquid such as chicken soup]. You'll be thirsty and you'll urinate easily." Each statement should be said three times.

- Establish a supportive doctor/patient relationship. Do this by asking all the questions you have, asking a nurse or anesthesiologist to say the healing statements, and making sure all your needs are met.

A pilot study done at Beth Israel Deaconess Medical Center found that hospitalized patients who were **not** going for surgery who used Peggy Huddleston's guided imagery tape for twenty minutes twice a day had a reduction in anxiety, used less pain medication and experienced an improvement in heart rate variability. An unpublished study found that forty-four patients going in for total knee replacement who used Peggy Huddleston's book and relaxation tape, and took her one hour workshop, were more calm the day of surgery and left the hospital 1.3 days sooner than controls. (See Peggy Huddleston's website, listed in "Resources," for information on this study.)

You can do these steps on your own by reading the book and using the relaxation CD, tape, or MP3 file. Some hospitals offer surgery-preparation classes based on the book, or you can find a health practitioner to lead you through a one-hour consultation by calling Huddleston's office. You can buy *Prepare for Surgery, Heal Faster* online. (For more information, turn to "Resources," at the back of the book.)

Following this program or using guided imagery techniques can help you feel more positive about an upcoming surgery. Although numerous studies have shown that patients who have positive attitudes about their operation have better surgical outcomes, there isn't much information available on preparing your mind for surgery. This book and audio program is one option. Meditation, which includes guided imagery and visualization, can be another way to prepare for an operation; to learn more about starting a practice, see Chapter 6, "Practices for the Mind."

Post-Surgical Life

After you have surgery, you'll need time to heal. You can complete some of Huddleston's surgery preparation tools post-operatively, as well:

- Practice relaxation. Use the *Prepare for Surgery, Heal Faster* relaxation CD, tape, or MP3 file. Alternatively, follow another guided imagery/visualization audio tape to take you into a state of relaxation for twenty minutes, twice a day.
- Visualize your healing. You can again use Huddleston's audio guide, or try using another guided imagery/visualization audio program for twenty minutes, twice a day.
- Have a supportive doctor/patient relationship. You might wonder if your scar is healing correctly or if the amount of pain you are feeling is appropriate. Ask your doctor any questions you have, and keep the lines of communication open.

It's important to take time to heal, asking family and friends to help care for you. A commitment to your post-operative rehabilitation program will also make your surgical outcomes as good as possible. Of course, surgery is just one piece of the puzzle. You may have pain and discomfort even after you fully heal from surgery. Trying other avenues to healing and pain relief can be beneficial. Read about other therapies, bodyworks, and exercise programs in this book. One or more of them might be a good fit for your lifestyle and your specific knee issue.

RESOURCES

Acufinder. www.acufinder.org

American Academy of Orthopaedic Surgeons. orthoinfo.aaos.org

American Academy of Physical Medicine and Rehabilitation. www.aapmr.org

American Board of Medical Specialties. 866-ASK-ABMS (275-2267). www.abms.org

American College of Sports Medicine. www.acsm.org

American Heart Association. www.americanheart.org

American Medical Society for Sports Medicine. 913-327-1415. www.amssm.org

The American Orthopaedic Society for Sports Medicine. 847-292-4900. www.sportsmed.org

American Osteopathic Association. 800-621-1773. www.osteopathic.org

American Physical Therapy Association. www.moveforwardpt.com

American Society for the Alexander Technique. 800-473-0620. www.alexandertech.org

American Society of Clinical Hypnosis. 630-980-4740. www.asch.net

The Arthritis Foundation. www.arthritis.org

Balanced Body Pilates. 800-745-2837. www.pilates.com

Benson-Henry Institute for Mind–Body Medicine. 617-643-6090. www.massgeneral.org/bhi/

Center for Mindfulness in Medicine, Health Care, and Society. 508-856-2656. www.umasssmed.edu/cfm

Cincinnati Children's Hospital Sports Medicine Biodynamics Center. www.cincinnatichildrens.org/sportsmed

ConsumerLab.com. www.consumerlab.com

ErgoMe. www.ergome.com

Feldenkrais Guild of North America. 800-775-2118. www.feldenkrais.com

Hellerwork Structural Integration/Hellerwork International. 714-873-6131. www.hellerwork.com

Huddleston, Peggy. 800-726-4173. www.HealFaster.com

International Association of Structural Integration. 877-843-4274. www.structuralintegration.org

Massage Today. www.massagetoday.com

The Mayo Clinic. www.mayoclinic.com

McKenzie Method. 800-635-8380. www.mckenziemdt.org/index_us.cfm

National Center for Complementary and Alternative Medicine. nccam.nih.gov

National Certification Board for Therapeutic Massage & Bodywork. 800-296-0664. www.ncbtmb.org

National Certification Commission for Acupuncture and Oriental Medicine. 904-598-1005. www.nccaom.org

Neutral Posture, Inc. 800-446-3746. www.igoergo.com

PEPS (Prevent injury, Enhance Performance) Program, created by the Santa Monica ACL Prevention Project. www.aclprevent.com

PNBConditioning. 206-441-2435; 425-451-1241. www.pnb.org/PNBSchool/PNBConditioning

Prescott, Cathy. www.yogawithCathy.com

Pujari, M.D., Astrid. www.pujaricenter.com

The Rolf Institute of Structural Integration. 800-530-8875. www.rolf.org

STOTT PILATES. 800-910-0001. www.stottpilates.com

Stretch Break. www.paratec.com

TheraSound. 717-582-4914/(532-7686). www.therasound.com

The Transcendental Meditation Program. 888-LEARN-TM. www.tm.org

Yoga Alliance Membership. 888-921-YOGA (9642). www.yogaalliance.org

Yoga Journal. www.yogajournal.com

BIBLIOGRAPHY

Benson, Herbert and Miriam Z. Klipper. *The Relaxation Response*. HarperCollins: New York, 2000.

Berthiaume, M-J, J-P Raynauld, J. Martel-Pelletier, F. Labonté, G. Beaudoin, D. A. Bloch, D. Choquette, B. Haraoui, R. D. Altman, M. Hochberg, J. M. Meyer, G. A. Cline, and J-P Pelletier. "Meniscal Tear and Extrusion are Strongly Associated with Progression of Symptomatic Knee Osteoarthritis as Assessed by Quantitative Magnetic Resonance Imaging." *Annals of the Rheumatic Diseases* 64 (2005): 556–563. (http://ard.bmj.com/cgi/content/abstract/64/4/556)

Blonstein, J. "Control of Swelling in Boxing Injuries." *Practitioner* 203 (1960): 206.

Byström, Sven E. G., Svend Erik Mathiassen, and Charlotte Fransson-Hall. "Physiological Effects of Micropauses in Isometric Handgrip Exercise." *European Journal of Applied Physiology and Occupational Physiology,* 63, no. 6 (December 2004): 405–411.

Duke University. *The Duke Encyclopedia of New Medicine: Conventional and Alternative Medicine for All Ages*. London: Rodale Books International, 2006.

Fu, F. H., et al. "Current Trends in Anterior Cruciate Ligament Reconstruction." *American Journal of Sports Medicine* 28, no.1 (January 2000): 123–130.

Goldberg, R. J., and J. Katz. "A Meta-Analysis of the Analgesic Effects of Omega-3 Polyunsaturated Fatty Acid Supplementation for Inflammatory Joint Pain." *Pain* 129, no. 1–2 (May 2007): 210–23.

Halpern, Brian, with Laura Tucker. *The Knee Crisis Handbook: Understanding Pain, Preventing Trauma, Recovering from Injury, and Building Healthy Knees for Life*. New York: LifeTime Media, Inc., 2003.

Heil, Nick. "The Owner's Manual: Your Knees." *Outside Magazine,* September 2006.

Huddleston, Peggy. *Prepare for Surgery, Heal Faster: A Guide of Mind–Body Techniques,* 2nd ed. Cambridge: Angel River Press, 2007.

Johnson, Jim. *Treat Your Own Knees: Simple Exercises to Build Strength, Flexibility, Responsiveness, and Endurance*. Alameda, California: Hunter House Inc., Publishers, 2003.

Kabat-Zinn, Jon. *Full Catastrophe Living: Using the Wisdom of Your Body and Mind to Face Stress, Pain, and Illness*. New York: Delta, 2005.

Kirkley, Alexandra, Trevor B. Birmingham, Robert B. Litchfield, J. Robert Giffin, Kevin R. Willits, Cindy J. Wong, Brian G. Feagan, Allan Donner, Sharon H. Griffin, Linda M. D'Ascanio, Janet E. Pope, and Peter J. Fowler. "A Randomized Trial of Arthroscopic Surgery for Osteoarthritis of the Knee." *The New England Journal of Medicine* 359, no. 11 (September 2008): 1097–1107.

Little, Paul, George Lewith, Fran Webley, Maggie Evans, Angela Beattie, Karen Middleton, Jane Barnett, Kathleen Ballard, Frances Oxford, Peter Smith, Lucy Yardley, Sandra Hollinghurst, and Debbie Sharp. "Randomised Controlled Trial of Alexander Technique Lessons, Exercise, and Massage (ATEAM) for Chronic and Recurrent Back Pain." *British Medical Journal,* 337: a884 (2008). (www.bmj.com/cgi/content/full/337/aug19_2/a884)

Madison, Deborah. *Vegetarian Cooking for Everyone*. New York: Broadway Books, 2007.

Mayo Foundation for Medical Education and Research. *Mayo Clinic Book of Alternative Medicine*. New York: Time Inc., 2007.

McCall, Timothy. *Yoga as Medicine*. New York: Bantam Dell, 2007.

Morone, Natalia E., Carol M. Greco, and Debra K. Weiner. "Mindfulness Meditation for the Treatment of Chronic Low-Back Pain in Older Adults: A Randomized Controlled Pilot Study." *Pain* 134, no. 3 (February, 2008): 310–319.

Moseley, Bruce J., Kimberly O'Malley, Nancy J. Petersen, Terri J. Menke, Baruch A. Brody, David H. Kuykendall, John C. Hollingsworth, Carol M. Ashton, and Nelda P. Wray. "A Controlled Trial of Arthroscopic Surgery for Osteoarthritis of the Knee." *The New England Journal of Medicine* 347, no. 2 (2002): 81–88.

Olsen, Odd-Egil, Grethe Myklebust, Lars Engebretsen, Ingar Holme, and Roald Bahr. "Exercises to Prevent Lower Limb Injuries in Youth Sports: Cluster Randomised Controlled Trial." *British Medical Journal* 330:449 (February 2005).

Orme-Johnson, David W., Robert H. Schneider, Young D. Son, Sanford Nidich, and Zang-Hee Cho. "Neuroimaging of Meditation's Effect on Brain Reactivity to Pain." *NeuroReport* 17, no. 12 (August 2006): 1359–63.

Parker, Steve. *The Human Body Book: An Illustrated Guide to Its Structure, Function, and Disorders*. New York: DK Publishing, 2007.

Patrick, G. "The Effects of Vibroacoustic Music on Symptom Reduction." *IEEE Engineering in Medicine and Biology,* March–April 1999: 97–100.

Peters. David, Dr. and Kenneth R. Pelletier. *New Medicine: Complete Family Health Guide.* New York: DK Publishing, 2007.

Pizzorno, Joseph and Michael Murray. *Encyclopedia of Natural Medicine.* New York: Three Rivers Press, 1998.

Puetz, Timothy W., Sara S. Flowers, and Patrick J. O'Connor. "A Randomized Controlled Trial of the Effect of Aerobic Exercise Training on Feelings of Energy and Fatigue in Sedentary Young Adults with Persistent Fatigue." *Psychother Psychosom* 77, no. 3 (2008): 167–74.

Sokolove, Michael. "The Uneven Playing Field." *The New York Times*, May 11, 2008. (www.nytimes.com/2008/05/11/magazine/11Girls-t.html)

Stricker, Lauri Ann. *Pilates for the Outdoor Athlete.* Golden, Colorado: Fulcrum Publishing, 2007.

Tapadinhas, M. J., et al. "Oral Glucosamine Sulfate in the Management of Arthrosis: Report on a Multi-Centre Open Investigation in Portugal." *Pharmatherapeutica* 3 (1982): 157–68.

Toth, M., P.M. Wolski, J. Foreman, R.B. Davis, T. Delbanco, R.S. Phillips, and P. Huddleston. "A Pilot Study for a Randomized, Controlled Trial on the Effect of Guided Imagery in Hospitalized Medical Patients." *The Journal of Alternative and Complementary Medicine* 13, No. 2 (March 2007): 194–197.

INDEX